Hey Hey It's Me!

DISCOVER WHY YOU NEED TO CHANGE YOUR LANGUAGE
IF
YOU ARE EVER GOING TO DROP THAT WEIGHT PERMANENTLY!

Your Body is Your Vehicle
to Carry You Through Life.
So … Drive Carefully!

Hey Hey It's Me!

No More 'Trying' to 'Lose' Weight and No More 'Diets'

Cas Willow & Heather Richards

Foreword by Gordon Emmerson, PhD

"If you are ready to become more knowledgeable about a balanced life and body, you may want to take some time and read this book carefully."

Published in Australia by Tophon Press

Copyright © 2014 Cas Willow and Heather Richards

All rights reserved. No part of this book may be reproduced by any mechanical, photographic or electronic process, or in the form of a phonographic recording; nor may it be stored in a retrieval system, transmitted or otherwise copied for public or private use, other than for 'fair use' as brief quotation embodied in articles and reviews, without prior written permission of the publisher.

If you would like to do any of the above, please seek permission first by contacting us at http://HeyHeyItsMe.com or http://CasWillow.com

Disclaimer

The information provided in this book is designed to provide helpful information on the subjects discussed. This book is not meant to be used, nor should it be used, to diagnose or treat any medical condition. For diagnosis or treatment of any medical problem, consult your own physician. The publisher and authors are not responsible for any specific health or allergy needs that may require medical supervision and are not liable for any damages or negative consequences from any treatment, action, application or preparation, to any person reading or following the information in this book. References are provided for informational purposes only and do not constitute endorsement of any websites or other sources. Readers should be aware that the websites listed in this book may change.

Cover Design: Cre8ive Ideas
Interior Sketches: Sandra Lee
Typeset by BookPOD Pty Ltd

The poem 'I Am Me' by Virginia Satir – Used with permission of the Virginia Satir Global Network www.satirglobal.org. All rights reserved.

ISBN: 978-0-9925138-0-1 (paperback)

Also available as an Audio Book ISBN: 978-0-9925138-2-5 and eBook ISBN: 978-0-9925138-1-8

A Catalogue-in-Publication is available from the National Library of Australia.

Acknowledgements

We would both like to acknowledge and thank our many mentors and teachers who have guided and supported us over the years in many different ways. They have showed us and shared countless strategies, frameworks and insights into the understanding, developing and implementing of human behaviour, as well as amazing techniques and strategies to assist and guide people to move through change when change is uncomfortable and uncertain.

To the many diverse clients of CaS Therapy (ranging in age from teenagers through to those in their seventies and eighties) who have allowed us to share their journey and lifestyle change, we thank you. We are honoured, privileged and humbled to have been able to be a part of your decision to change your way of life to one of your choosing, one that is right and healthy for you, within your own standards and guidelines.

Special thanks to those members of our families who have supported, encouraged, accepted and believed in us. We thank you for your motivation, encouragement and consistent positivity.

A huge thank you to Noush, Phoebe, Tobias, Bert, John and Peppa for the belief and trust that you have invested daily in us and what we do. A big thank you to our dear friends and greatest supporters, who include Victoria and Stacey. To the many special colleagues who have given so generously of their time, offering support, suggestions and opportunities, we sincerely thank you.

We also thank and acknowledge each other individually. We realise that we both have unique and amazing skills, drive and knowledge. However, together we are a dynamic team, supporting, encouraging and appreciating the strengths and weaknesses that we both possess.

Finally, we want to acknowledge our amazing parts, our weak and childish parts that wish to have fun, our strong and intellectual parts that strive to achieve, our loving and caring parts that want to help others and the parts of us that recognise the global obesity issue is a choice that needs to be addressed one person at a time. And the parts of us that believe in ourselves, our message and the need to share our knowledge with others.

Contents

Acknowledgements v

Foreword xi

About the Authors xiii

Preface xix
    From Tank to Sports Car xix

Important Note to Readers xxi
    Resources We Suggest xxii

Introduction and How to Read This Book 1
    The 7 Life Steps for a healthy lifestyle 1
    Setting steps for life 2

Chapter 1: Living a Healthy Lifestyle – Weight Management – a Lifestyle Choice 17
    A brief overview of what this book is about 17
    Weight loss and language 23
    Weight management and motivation 27
    Self-reflective questions for weight management 32

Chapter 2: Purpose – What is Behind Your Decision? 35
    Examining what is behind your decision to manage your weight 35
    Discovering your purpose in life – what drives you? 43
    The CaS Therapy 7 Core Principles 48
    Reasons you may hold on to weight subconsciously – secondary gains 49

Chapter 3: 'Try' and 'Hope' 57
- What is your relationship with food? 57
- Feeding the mouth and the mind 60
- How motivated are you to drop weight and gain better health? 62
- Why you eat – uncovering unhealthy associations 62
- Practising mindful eating 67
- Being one with the body 71

Chapter 4: Diet Versus a Healthy Lifestyle 77
- What do you say to yourself when you hear the word 'diet'? 77
- Food as fuel – the sports car analogy 81
- Eating to live versus living to eat 84

Chapter 5: Eating and Your Emotions 91
- The emotional connection with food 91
- Practising feeling your emotions 96
- Food addictions 99
- NLP exercises to practise 102

Chapter 6: The Role of Nutrition in Health 107
- The ABCs of good nutrition 107
- Planting the seeds 110
- Learning how to eat REAL nourishing food 112
- Living and eating healthy as a lifestyle choice 116

Chapter 7: The Clean Slate Process 123
- Identifying limiting beliefs that serve no purpose 123
- What is it you believe when it comes to weight management? 126
- What is the belief behind this? 127
- Converting those reasons to positive statements 133

Chapter 8: Acceptance and the Body 141
- Taking responsibility for where you are in this moment 141
- Loving yourself NOW– no matter what shape or size 148
- Finding the motivation you need to move forward 150

    Body acceptance exercise 154

Chapter 9: Setting Goals and Envisioning the NEW YOU 159
    Setting the goals 159
    Changing your self-image through future pacing 164
    What will you look like? 164
    Imagine – what will you feel like? 166

Chapter 10: The Scanner 173
    Learning to read the body's signals 173
    Being appreciative of the body 177
    Activating your other senses 179

Chapter 11: The Remote Control 183
    Dialling down your hunger 183
    How do you know when you are really hungry? 185
    How do you know when you are satiated? 187
    Dealing with hunger 188
    The remote control in action 189

Chapter 12: Self-Hypnosis Exercise 195
    What is self-hypnosis versus hypnosis? 195
    Brief background of hypnosis 197
    Brain wave frequencies – tapping into the Alpha state of mind 199
    A simple self-hypnosis exercise 201

Conclusion 209

References 213

Foreword

There have been myriads of approaches to weight management presented over the last few years, including physically aggressive techniques of stomach stapling and strange diets that espouse everything from large amounts of water, fat, protein, raw foods, and the list goes further and further.

The person with unwanted weight has been blamed for having the wrong set point, for being weak willed, and for being ignorant of what skinnier people know.

There have been other books that look at the psychology of weight loss, as does this book, but *Hey Hey It's Me! Lifestyle & Weight Management* presents a collage of weight management approaches without any fad diets or physically demanding techniques. It does not ask the reader to take pills or ascribe to the latest craze of oil or tonic. Seven Steps and 32 Activities are presented so the reader can learn and practise techniques that may be helpful to them to gain empowerment in focusing, healing and taking on a healthy lifestyle that will result in a healthy weight.

This book sneaks up on you. When reading it there may be times when it seems like a lot of disconnected information, but reading it is an education. As you read, a larger picture begins to come into focus, a picture of a whole life approach.

Weight management is not something that can be captured in a few short buzz words or phrases. In order to change a way of life it takes a holistic understanding of what is a healthy life. It requires becoming educated about a myriad of things that can impact upon a healthy diet. The authors of this book are clear that diet does not mean anything crash, it means knowledge and lifestyle.

If you are ready to become more knowledgeable about a balanced life and body, you may want to take some time and read this book carefully.

Gordon Emmerson, PhD

Author: *Healthy Parts, Happy Self*
Ego State Therapy
Advanced Skills and Interventions in Therapeutic Counseling
Resource Therapy Primer

About the Authors

A little about Cas Willow

Cas was the youngest of five girls before two more half-sisters came along, making her one of seven children. Cas was a target of schoolyard bullying and painful name calling, such as 'Freckle Face Fatty "R" Buckle', by students and adults, including teachers. This reinforced a low opinion of self, setting the foundations for a dysfunctional belief system and low self-worth.

At home the children were often made to eat low grade food and piles of mashed potato for dinner to fill them up. Hungry and experiencing hunger pains, the girls were often sent off to bed. Meanwhile, the adults dined on quality steaks and vegetables. Thus the cravings for food and love lingered.

Cas recalls times after school when she and two of her sisters would sneak inside the family home and eat food they were specifically told they were not allowed to eat. This set up patterns of secrets, sneaking and feeling not worthy of quality foods, which triggered the survival parts within Cas.

Naturally, this laid the foundation for Cas having experiences of food deprivation, leading to a desire to seek, want and crave foods that were ingrained as forbidden fruits. Eating and overeating at any opportunity that presented itself for comfort and subconsciously overcompensating as a protection, led to Cas becoming morbidly obese.

In order to escape the sadness of the family home, Cas married at a very young age. With that came freedom, followed by more uncontrolled desires to eat all of the food and treats that she had been deprived of (and not educated about) for many, many years.

It was in her early 20s that a very unhappy Cas, weighing around 132kg, began her journey. The start of the thought process of being overweight led to an unhealthy mental attitude that saw Cas drop to well below a healthy weight. However, with strong determination and a considerable amount of assistance, Cas chose a career in the helping profession and began her personal journey to happiness. Educating herself and having a burning desire to help others has steered Cas to become the remarkable therapist that she is today. Cas has not only been able to drop from the big young woman she was to a healthy weight range she has also been able to maintain her weight at less than half of that amount constantly throughout her adult life, supporting a healthy lifestyle pathway.

Cas and Heather together run a successful therapy centre, where they assist many people who want to be helped with their own personal weight management journey. Cas hopes that the revelation of just a small part of her personal journey inspires and encourages others to make their own decision to change their lifestyle. This book is based on their weight management and lifestyle program and aims to help, guide and arm those seeking assistance with the tools that are necessary to make the required changes. Life begins with you, right now, today! You can have the life you choose.

And a little about Heather Richards too.

Heather was brought up in what would be considered a normal family environment, Mum, Dad and five children. Her father worked hard to bring in the income, whilst her mother stayed home to keep house and look after the children.

Being the fourth born into the household after three boys brought with it some of its own problems and underlying issues. These were compounded by ongoing comments and remarks, such as not being planned and being an accident, which also bandied around to her sister arriving into the family many years later. This left long-lasting effects of not being wanted and a yearning to feel wanted, to belong and be accepted.

Heather would like it to be known, that she loves her parents and is extremely grateful for all they have done and supported her through in her life. She totally understands and accepts that any hurt, or pain is her own perception of any events or circumstances and no malice would ever have been the intention of either of her loving parents, who like many parents did their best to bring up their children in a safe, secure and loving environment.

Heather recalls her paternal grandmother as a rather large woman and was constantly programmed as a child that she too would grow up to be big just like her. It is true that children do not come with a manual (well not yet; we plan on writing one with regard to programming with positives throughout the developmental years), however, they are very much programmed by their environment and the beliefs and patterns that they are introduced to as children.

Because she was a girl, sports and exercise were not considered as important. That was something the boys were encouraged to partake in by Dad (for example football and cricket). Mum was not interested in sport so it was not something that was required or expected. Through the schooling years and due to other things that occurred throughout Heather's childhood, her confidence levels and self-esteem were really quite low. Whilst she believes she covered this on the surface quite well, she would go to great lengths to avoid sports and change rooms at as many opportunities as she could. It was the other childhood incidents that Heather, through her education later in life, realised were most likely the reasons behind her subconsciously carrying a barrier of protection around her by carrying a certain amount of weight.

As every child, Heather sought love, attention and affection. Often the attention came with (what she believes was unintentional and a result of a lack of human behavioural education) emotional conditions. Comments like 'If you do this, you can have this' or 'If you run this message, you can have that' were commonplace. Often the reward was chocolates, lollies, soft drink or ice-cream – therefore, programming her as a child to associate sweets with the warm and fuzzy feelings of love and attention from adults.

Looking back now and seeing photos of herself in her early 20s when she was a size 8 or 10, she can see just how trim and slim she was. However, Heather's recollection of that time and her perception of herself was that her size was still big.

She has many memories of members of her family commenting on her weight, comments like 'Oh you have been in a good paddock' or 'You are one of the short, round members of the family' or whilst being held down and tickled her top coming up and hearing comments of disgust. Sure, they may seem like harmless enough and yes, the intention may have been in jest; however, ongoing comments like these just re-enforce and compound suggestions that in turn the mind believes to be true and as we know, what the mind believes the mind can conceive. Even in later years and right to this day it is commonplace for members of the family to comment on weight as a part of the initial welcoming greeting and this is a common occurrence within many families. Unfortunately, often the people commenting have no awareness of the long-term impacts of their constant insensitive comments.

Whilst Heather has never seen herself as obese, she has certainly struggled with the thought process behind the weight that she has carried for her entire life, even when weight was clearly not an issue for her. However, her programming was that she was big and would grow up to be big and, therefore, that is how she saw herself.

Little, what appeared to be harmless, sayings experienced as a child like 'Sticks and stones will break your bones, but names can never hurt you' are so untrue. Research shows that emotional torment is just as hurtful, painful and long lasting and often more so than physical torment.

Heather has come to a lot of realisations over the last few years as she has studied human behaviours. She has realised that a lot of behaviours in bringing up children in what were considered normal, nice, average type families, may lay a lot of insecure foundations on an emotional level for many children, who bring those habits and behaviours with them into adulthood.

Heather and Cas team together to compile this book.

Heather and Cas see this book as a healthy lifestyle manual based on their successful weight management program. If they are able to help and assist people with their weight struggle or have parents stop and think before they place conditions on giving their children the 'unconditional' love and attention that every child brought into this world deserves, then the task of writing this book and sharing their experiences and knowledge has been worth the journey.

Preface

From Tank to Sports Car

Our analogy, our metaphor – 'The Roadmap to Living a Healthy Lifestyle'
The Roadmap to Living a Healthy Lifestyle is about the vehicle being your vessel that carries you through life. Think about what a body requires to function effectively day in, day out, seven days a week, week after week, month after month and year after year. Your heart continues to beat for years and years, if that is what destiny has in place for you. If you do not take care of your body and your mind, then the body and mind slowly whittle away and break down because they eventually wear out. Some bodies live longer than others, we just need to ensure that we do the best we can to take care of what we are originally given. The vehicle, being your body, also requires a certain amount of maintenance to keep it running effectively, day in and day out. This analogy focuses on you being the vehicle, tapping into the vehicle that is driving you on the roads, transporting you through bumps, hurdles, around obstacles, experiencing experiences, and enduring adventures, driving you through to where your destiny lies. So make sure you pick the type of vehicle that suits you best, so you can learn to drive on the road to your chosen destination. You may want a sporty vehicle, so you choose the colour and away you go as you read and follow this book intensively.

Whatever your size, shape or status, you can transform yourself into whatever vehicle you choose and ensure that you have a vehicle that drives the body to its destination in a way that you choose. Your body is your vehicle, the vehicle that drives you through this journey of life, and you choose your destination and the pathways that you wish to travel from your own internal and external maps that are presented to you throughout your life. What you do and how you look after your vehicle is determined by where you are at right now. If you want your vehicle to happily and peacefully carry you through life, we need to ensure it is filled with adventures, excitement and the correct fuel, learning the complete way to be true to yourself and to do what matters most, what is important to you, as you are here in this lifetime, living the life that is significant to you NOW.

Let's do a reality check now. You want to change, obviously, that is why you are reading this book, so what we are hearing is that you are currently not happy with your lifestyle and you want to be different. Is that right? If the answer is 'yes', then keep reading. If the answer is 'no', then check in with self to see what it is you actually desire.

You picked up this book and have obviously started to flick through it, so something is happening within your mind and your body right now that perhaps this book could be helpful and useful for you in some way.

You see, when you sit in a vehicle you usually have a destination in mind. You turn the vehicle on and you then take off towards that destination. The mind drives the vehicle knowing where you are headed. So if your mind does not know where you are going within your life, how is the mind meant to know where to go? Does it make sense that you need to let the mind know exactly what it is you want and what your needs are, so you can drive the mind to form the actions to achieve all that you desire?

How committed to self are you?
On a scale of 1 to 10, how much do you really want to change, to do different and live that healthy lifestyle you want? How much of your life are you willing to put into action, to improve your health? You can read all the books you like, learn everything you want and need to, however, remember, unless you **commit to action**, start the process, nothing will change. This book identifies what matters, what is useful and helpful and empowers you to make those changes that you have decided to action.

So if you are ready, let us begin our journey together.

Important Note to Readers

As with any weight, health, fitness or lifestyle program, readers are advised to consult a physician before making any major change in diet, exercise routine or anything else in their life.

This book is not just another diet and weight loss book. If that was all it was, we could sum it up in three very short chapters:

Chapter 1: Drink More Water
Chapter 2: Eat Less Food
Chapter 3: Do More Exercise.

Our book is based on the tried and tested system we use in our weight management and lifestyle program at our therapy centre in Melbourne, where we explore feelings and hidden emotions behind why we eat the way we do and look into the old patterns and beliefs that we formed as we grew up.

We then guide you through the steps that make our program so successful for so many people.

The key is: You really do need to be ready to change and do the things that are necessary to bring about that change. You need to '**commit to action**'.

We believe that everybody at some time or another has issues relating to something or someone in their life. If these issues are having an unhelpful or negative impact on your life, then it may be time to seek the assistance of a professional therapist. If you would like the assistance of a CaS Therapy professional therapist, then please feel free to contact the centre directly. Please remember that a book is not, and cannot replace, a therapist.

If you are ready to do the work, let us begin.

Resources We Suggest

In order to complete some of the activities throughout the book, we would like to suggest some tools that may be helpful and useful to you. However, you may decide to keep everything in the mind, and we would like to encourage you to do what suits you and works best for you as this is all about you.

- The 'Note It Book' ('the NIB'). You will notice throughout references to 'pop it in the NIB'. Your NIB can be a standard exercise writing book, a sketch book, a book with an eye-catching cover, or it can be one of convenience. Whatever you choose, ensure it suits you best, as this book will soon become akin to your best friend. So stay focused and remember to note it in the NIB. Notice and observe any thoughts, feelings, behaviours, patterns, language and anything else that you may NOTICE and put it in the 'NIB'. This may include what you notice about the food you eat, when you eat and for what purpose you believe you are eating, at that time. All you need to do is add some headings which can help you along the way.

Some of the headings we suggest to get you started are:

DATE	TIME	THOUGHTS	FEELINGS	PATTERNS
ACTIONS	SENSES	WHO	WHAT	WHEN
NOTICED	WHERE	HOW	STRENGTHS	NEW EXPERIENCE

- A4 & A3 sheets of paper (including coloured paper if that suits you best).

- Crayons, pens or even coloured textas or markers. This is not about drawing a Mona Lisa; this is all about expression, exploration and discovery.

- An audio player of some kind and music if you so choose.

- Private space/area to complete the set activities that incorporate your life-changing decisions. Your beautiful voice and all your senses.

Introduction and How to Read This Book

The 7 Life Steps for a healthy lifestyle

The following seven steps explain everything that the CaS Therapy programs contain to make those changes that you have '*committed to action*'. These steps are called the 'Life Steps' of a person's cycle within their timeline. These steps are all entwined within the imprinting stage. Building all the seven steps to construct strong foundations both in the mind and body. Living, being, thinking, feeling and eating healthy every day, before long these steps for life become a natural organic process.

This natural organic process forms the true imprint and your '**Weigh of Life**'. In order for you to be the one standing on your own pedestal in your own life, worshipping your own body and mind, each of the following steps needs to be mastered and respected.

The CaS Therapy '**A Weigh of Life**' CD is available if you would like some further assistance to help you move into living a healthy life:

It is available in Australia from our website www.CasWillow.com/products/a-weigh-of-life (in Australia only), or from

http://tinyurl.com/amazon-weighoflife (where shipping is available worldwide via Amazon).

Setting steps for life

Complete the seven steps for life by working through each individual step and committing to all of them to move you forward. Allow a realistic time frame that suits you and ensure that what you are asking of your body and mind is relevant and attainable specific to your needs and wants. Remember to NOTICE and note in the NIB.

Each step guides and supports you at your own pace, allowing time for changes to occur. Each step gives you the tools to permanently imprint and action the roadmap for life, an exciting and easy step by step process to action the change.

As we talk about the seven steps, you may notice that each has its own little world. What that actually means is, even though each step connects to another, you live within that step until it is fully completed.

Each of the chapters cumulates to a step, taking you through experiential exercises and activities that assist such a change. Know that each individual step is required to be completed and mastered before moving on to the next. If you arrive at a step that does not feel right just yet, then simply return to the step prior and run through it again. Remember, there is no rush or time limit; this is your '**weigh of life**', the '**weigh of life**' you have chosen to live each day.

As you make your way through each chapter, work with the steps and tick off each activity as you progress through the book. You are in control and this is a process to be undertaken at your own pace.

Step 1 Laying the Foundation

Foundations are important in any structure or plan. When planning to build a home, for example, one must first list what needs to be included. One then develops a plan and, like

Relevant Chapters

1. Living a Healthy Lifestyle
2. Purpose
3. 'Try' and 'Hope'

with all homes, the correct foundations must be dug out and laid, so they are strong enough to build a solid structure upon to last a lifetime.

For Step 1, take the time to really explore and reflect through Chapters 1, 2 and 3, and for Step 2, explore and reflect on Chapters 4 and 5 before continuing to Step 3. Complete honestly and openly all activities at your own pace. Remember, we are laying the fundamentals, so we need to ensure that the foundation is strong and prepared for all that is required to be built on top of those strong foundations. Gather those pens, crayons, coloured texta markers and your NIB, ready to participate fully and effectively, and really commit to the new you.

A lifestyle choice is yours for the taking...

What language is in the now for you?

Have you completed the activity – Self-reflective questions?

Are you ready to live healthy, be healthy, eat healthy and think healthy?

What have you chosen to do about your new lifestyle and how and who can help you?

- ☐ Activity 1 – Self-reflective questions for weight management
- ☐ Activity 2 – Reasons why my subconscious chooses to hold my excess weight
- ☐ Activity 3 – Reasons to do different
- ☐ Activity 4 – My life purpose
- ☐ Activity 5 – Exercise to reveal life purpose
- ☐ Activity 6 – Feeding the mouth and the mind
- ☐ Activity 7 – Meeting five needs
- ☐ Activity 8 – Thought stopping band

Step 2 Resetting Language

The word 'language' covers all aspects of communication from verbal to body, to symbols and codes. Communication pathways can only be interpreted through the

Relevant Chapters
4. Diet vs a Healthy Lifestyle
5. Eating and Your Emotions

eyes of the receiver. Remember, how we communicate and how we actually transmit the information we want to share could possibly be translated into something perhaps you do not really mean. The intended communication could become lost in translation.

SENDER	Messages can become lost in translation through:	RECEIVER
When we send a message like: *'You need to cook the cake at 180°C or it will burn,'* what the sender is actually saying is: *'Cakes burn if they are cooked at a higher temperature.'*	• Interpretation • Beliefs • Morals • Faulty systems • Experiences • Learning • External influences • Mind altering drugs • Perceptions • Half stories • Sensitive thoughts	The receiver could translate the message from the sender as: *'What are you saying, I can't cook?'* rather than: *'The cake is sensitive and requires a stable average temperature, nothing more.'*

The whole communication process that language is compiled of requires a sender and a receiver, even if the sender and the receiver is you, or the same person:

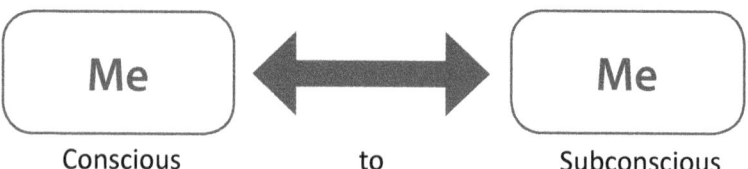

Me — Conscious   to   Me — Subconscious

The conscious mind is the analysis of the brain often working overtime as it filters, perceives and interprets and sometimes may not even be on the right track. The subconscious mind is black or white. It does not interpret and it is very clear within its thinking, even if it does not make sense to your conscious mind. The subconscious mind holds the beliefs, values and patterns of behaviour that contribute to your everyday behaviours.

Language needs to be:

- Useful Information
- Relevant
- Clear & precise
- Directional
- Considerate
- Informative
- Specific
- Focused
- Purposeful
- Adequate

Language is full of semantic meanings which can be very powerful. Semantics contain the analysis of the actual meaning of words through their combination in a sentence or story. These words can be the honesty of communication between sender and receiver. This simply means that how precise and clear we are with the message we are communicating (sending) determines the clarity at the end for the receiver. Step 2 defines the space in between the sender and the receiver as the total resetting of language.

Each activity in Step 2, works through the initial stages of the wonders of communicating. Continue to complete the following activities:

☐ Activity 9 – Diet vs healthy lifestyle
☐ Activity 10 – Healthy lifestyle exercise
☐ Activity 11 – Learning and exploring emotions
☐ Activity 12 – Important NLP step

Step 3 Planting the Seeds

As we climb the steps we will gain a greater understanding of language and how the conscious and subconscious communicate, and

Relevant Chapters
6. The Role of Nutrition

the importance of learning from the past, to use those learnings in the present to move into the future.

This step focuses on the planting of new ideas, behaviours and thoughts, so that new and improved behaviours and thinking patterns manifest you into the person of your choice. Learning about nutrition and what food actually does for you can take you to places that perhaps you have never previously been. This step helps you to change your relationship with food, bringing that relationship to a whole new level. Each action taken, even reading and working through these steps, is part of the 'journey of a thousand miles' in your new healthy life.

Affirmations are a powerful collection of words and meanings that create the platform for purpose and direction to do different. Ensure that by now you have made room for the seeds you have planted in the garden of the mind to grow and prosper.

The Food Pyramid is part of learning about where food fits into our daily life. Our body and mind need to refuel and re-energise so they can function to the best of their abilities. Your food relationship can only grow and flourish to an innovative dimension.

Remember to continue to check off the activities as you proceed through the book.

☐ Activity 13 – Eating in a healthy manner
☐ Activity 14 – Food Pyramid

Introduction and How to Read This Book

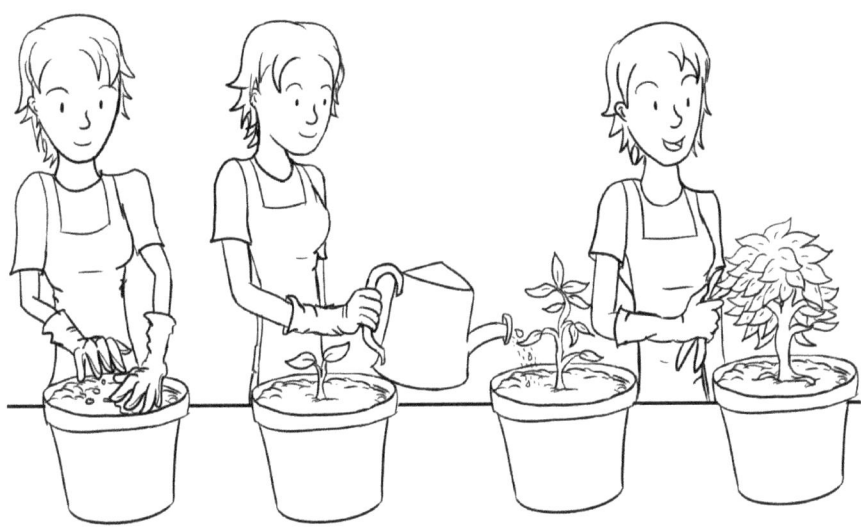

Step 4 Cleaning the Slate

This is such a magical step. This step is to ensure that you have gathered your learnings and released your old thoughts, habits, feelings, behaviours

Relevant Chapters

7. The Clean Slate Process

and patterns so that you are now ready to create the lifestyle of your choosing.

As you work through Step 4, visualise the road. You stand in the middle. You have chosen a pathway and a direction. Know that whatever obstacles or blocks that may appear along your chosen path, you already have everything you need to keep you on track, driving forward in the direction of your goal. So, direct your eyes forward on the road as you begin this journey.

Be sure to be totally honest with your answers to yourself. This is the time for your mind to connect to the motivational drive to eat, feel, think and be healthy. Activity 16 will assist with the '**FLiPiT**' attitude that will lead to permanent change.

> # FLiPiT
>
> * F – Free – The Old Words
> * L – Lift – The New Words
> * i – Increase – The meaning of the words
> * P – Positive – Reinforcement
> * i – Include – Real truths
> * T – Transform – anything & everything

The **FLiPiT** attitude can be incorporated into everything you say and do. Stay focused on the task at hand. Now you are ready for the clean slate exercise. Take your time and know that you can repeat this step as often as you need.

☐ Activity 15 – Underlying associations

☐ Activity 16 – List 10 reasons

☐ Activity 17 – 10 positive affirmations

☐ Activity 18 – Clean slate exercise

Step 5 Imprinting Stage

Taking responsibility for where you are at this very moment is a vital component of the imprinting process. Like the true image of tattooing, we want it to be permanent despite whatever has been there previously.

Relevant Chapters

8. Acceptance and the Body
9. Setting Goals and Envisioning the New You

These two chapters assist with this step for the 'imprint' to leave a mark. The chapters cover goals setting and working with the SMART system to set goals. Okay now...

It's time to do it!

Commit to self a time each day and week that incorporates the 'Acceptance Exercise'. You can start by writing your own way to accept and make room for who you are from the inside.

An example could be:

'The Acceptance of Action Poem'

> I accept who I am, I commit to action to do different, I am free to be me. I have made the choice to respect and make room for who I am. I free myself from any attachment and threads from my past views and beliefs upon who I am. I welcome what my body does, the role of my arms, hands, legs and feet and all that my body continues to do each day. I am unique and I am an individual.
>
> I am free to be the person I choose to be
> I am (*add your name here*)

Now you can utilise this 'Acceptance of Action' poem, or 'I Am Me' by Virginia Satir (1975) in Chapter 8, or even create your own. Whatever you choose, be precise and truthful as this is all about you and you are important and what matters.

The values and beliefs section helps you identify what is truly important to you, so you can have the directional pathway that keeps you moving. We mean moving in the literal way, with the rhythm of life, enjoying the experiences that life has to offer.

Step 5 incorporates goal setting which steers the vehicle on the road to the destination that one chooses to drive.

Part of the imprinting stage is to ensure that you follow the '**CARREZ**' model. This model provides the framework for you to refer back to and recheck that you are active whilst you are committing to action to ensure that you live an extraordinary lifestyle.

```
           CARREZ
                        H
        C – Commit      E
                        A
        A – Accept      L
                        T
                        H
        R – Respect     Y

        R – Reflect     L
                        I
        E – Embrace     V
                        I
                        N
        Z – Zone        G
```

COMMIT to action is the aid that assists with the physical and emotional movement to ensure that each day you are living those choices you make according to your values and beliefs.

ACCEPT is making room for all the hurt and pain experiences and knowledge that flow through into your daily life so you can make room for living the way you choose to live.

RESPECT follows the pathway of self-respect and respecting others which leads into the areas of self-awareness and owning a responsibility to you to make those chosen changes.

REFLECT is the vital stage to ensure that you stay on the self-awareness pathway to ensure growth and change, keeping you on track and living true to your values.

EMBRACE focuses on the new and the different, embracing new patterns and behaviours that you have put into place to bring about the change to live that new lifestyle.

ZONE brings you into the space to be focused and committed to action, living the lifestyle that you have chosen, being, feeling, eating, living and thinking healthy – a whole new way of being, to live an extraordinary life.

This is your time for you.

Remember to check through the **CARREZ** model to ensure that you are where you need to be. You can always alter the goals you have put in place. You have the power to control each directional pathway as you go through life.

- ☐ Activity 19 – Thanking body
- ☐ Activity 20 – Values and beliefs
- ☐ Activity 21 – Moving the body
- ☐ Activity 22 – Body acceptance
- ☐ Activity 23 – My SMART goal
- ☐ Activity 24 – Imagining the new you

You have now reached a critical section. Ensure that you are clear and confident within the space in which you currently sit prior to moving on to Step 6.

Go through the checklist!

If all the items are checked off then proceed. If not, then NOW is the time to STOP and ensure all the activities have been completed.

Step 6 Resetting the Internal Dialogue System

This step guides you through the internal dialogue that constantly influences your thoughts, feelings and behaviours. The most important element in Step 6 is the awareness factor.

Relevant Chapters

10. The Scanner
11. The Remote Control

Make the time to do Step 6 wherever and whenever you need to as this step will come into play more often than you think. This step will become an automatic system that operates at the deeper level.

Discovering and learning to read your own body signals takes time. NOW, we want you to do something right at this moment:

Close your eyes and notice what you hear, smell, taste, touch, and then open your eyes and notice what you see first.

Write this down in your NIB.

When you have completed this activity, you are ready to move on to Chapter 10. If you have not completed this activity, then stop. Spend some time now and master tapping into your true senses. Remember, this is not a race and you are worth the time. It is time well spent on your very own personal development and growth.

The two chapters associated with Step 6 increase your self-awareness and empower your senses to work with you and for you, creating a true 'Body Scan' image.

This '**Body Scan**' incorporates the cousin chapter the '**Remote Control**'. The **remote control** is simply there for you to ensure that those parts of you are empowered to say 'no' and to alter and change everyday occurances associated with feelings and thoughts. Enjoy and have fun using these two amazing personal growth tools.

Introduction and How to Read This Book

- ☐ Activity 25 – Tapping into self-awareness
- ☐ Activity 26 – Tapping into the senses
- ☐ Activity 27 – The Body Scan
- ☐ Activity 28 – Where are you now?
- ☐ Activity 29 – Remote Control in action

Step 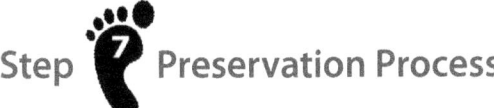 Preservation Process

This last step is covered in the final chapter and is designed to ensure that any changes you make have the space to be permanent. This step

Relevant Chapters

12. Self-Hypnosis Exercise

enables the complete structure and process to be configured which then becomes stored in the preservation stage of living. We permanently lock in what works, what is useful, our choices and directions, as well as our altered thoughts and behaviours, creating the entire roadmap that is unique and suitable for you.

CRAN
* Check
* Reflect
* Adjust
* Nurture

The preservation process is a simple and easy system that can be completed on a monthly time frame. All you need to do is use the **CRAN** safeguarding system. The **CRAN** safeguards you to living a healthy lifestyle that you choose and requires simple, regular attention, just like brushing your teeth, for example. If you do not brush your teeth then the consequences can cost you dearly and can cause several health problems. Remember what is important to you. ☺

By the time you reach Chapter 12 you have completed all the work to bring about a whole new way of thinking, feeling and doing. You will have created the life you want and who you want to be, who you want to look like and what you want to feel like. Is that what is important?

Of course, this is why you are here on this journey. So, in the preservation process, applying the **CRAN** is quite simple and easy to implement into a regular routine.

Utilise the following template to apply your very own **CRAN** safeguard system.

Apply Preservation Process

C = Check
1. _____
2. _____
3. _____
4. _____

R = Reflect
1. _____
2. _____
3. _____
4. _____

A = Adjust

N = Nurture
_____
_____
_____

Remember, you have everything you need within the library of the mind. Let's make sure that you have mastered the self-hypnosis which incorporates affirmations into your everyday life.

Chapter 12 takes you on the journey of really discovering the power of the mind. It is your mind and you are in control.

- ☐ Activity 30 – Self-hypnosis
- ☐ Activity 31 – Affirmations
- ☐ Activity 32 – CRAN maintenance checklist

Congratulations! You have now completed the 32 activities that have you driving on the road and in the direction that you have chosen – Well done!

Chapter 1

Living a Healthy Lifestyle – Weight Management – a Lifestyle Choice

A brief overview of what this book is about

If you are tired of struggling with your weight, you are certainly not alone. The reality is that no matter what you do, the mathematical equation of weight management remains the same.

> What you eat – What you do = You!

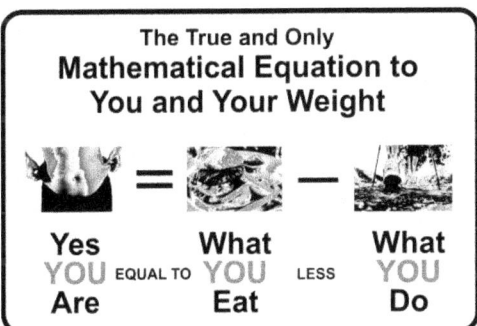

There is really nothing magical about this formula; it just simply is a mathematical fact.

The formula simply outlines that the body needs to balance all that goes in so it can come out in some way, either by energy or waste. The body only needs to consume small amounts of food and plenty of water to function effectively. Over time our stomachs stretch, which opens the doors for more food to be consumed. The reality is that the weight is there for a reason. Some of the questions we will ask you to ask yourself will be focused on what role food plays in your life and how it shapes what you think, feel and do. How much easier would life be if we did not have to struggle to lose weight, if we could easily live a healthy balanced life each and every day? You are going to find many answers to questions that may have just lain dormant. This book focuses on living a healthy life, which begins and is maintained within the mind.

First, let's mention 'diets'. They are not an effective long-term solution, often work short-term and never actually address the core issues behind why the weight is there in the first place. The object of this book is to help streamline the pathways of being healthy, living healthy, eating healthy, feeling healthy and thinking healthy.

In order for the weight to drip away, there is a part of you or many parts of you that need to want to change, that are willing to make the change to let go of the weight. Those parts need to work with other parts of the mind that really want the weight to drip away. How important is becoming a lower weight to you? If you have tried everything for the weight to drip away and have become fit, yet with little to no results, then keep reading as we are sure that there is a part of you that wants to 'do different', simply because you are continuing to read. By the time you complete this process and read through the upcoming chapters, you will have a much clearer idea of how your emotions affect the body, the mind and therefore, your weight.

You will notice that throughout this book we will continue to refer to three main therapies which we have found to be most effective when assisting with change: Counselling, Ego State Therapy and Hypnotherapy.

Chapter 1
Living a Healthy Lifestyle – Weight Management – a Lifestyle Choice

The 'counselling' process is about the counsellor supporting, assisting and guiding you to work through your issues, addressing your needs at your own pace, empowering you to strive and pursue your chosen pathway. Counselling is a confidential process primarily focused on empowering and enhancing the psychological well-being of people, thus enabling you to reach your full potential. Counselling is about helping people, exploring patterns and behaviours, identifying obstacles, learning developmental experiences and working with the learnings of the client, focusing on empowering them to live the life they choose (Geldard & Geldard, 2012).

Ego State Therapy 'is based on the premises that personality is composed of separate parts, rather than being a homogenous whole' (Emmerson, 2009, p. 1).

> These parts are called Ego States. We are always speaking or acting from one of our Ego States. For example, when we say 'Part of me wants to go out' that is one Ego State saying that it is ready to go out and enjoy the night. Then we may also say, 'But part of me would rather just stay home and laze around in my PJs watching television'. Clearly, that is another part that is ready to rest and relax in the comfort of our home. Each state has its power, strength, vulnerability, emotion, reason and behaviour. When we say, 'Part of me...,' we are talking from an Ego State. Our various states make our lives what they are today and in some instances, to improve our quality of life, we need to address the issues affecting some states. A state harbouring pain or discomfort can cause an unsettled and unwanted emotional reaction (CaSandh Pty. Ltd. & Richards, 2010).

Hypnosis is an altered state of consciousness that everybody experiences.

> Hypnotherapy, which is therapy under hypnosis, reaches the subconscious part of the mind where your beliefs, learnings, values, experiences, and memories lie. Hypnotherapy is an easy and gentle way for the mind and body to heal naturally. Hypnotherapy interacts with the conscious and the subconscious mind focusing on core

issues which can be addressed and where changes can occur on a more profound level. When a person enters into a 'hypnotic state' this term simply means that they have entered an 'altered state of consciousness'. The person is totally in control of self and continues to have an awareness of the whole hypnotherapy process (CaSandH Pty. Ltd., 2010).

Utilising these tools either together or individually can help undo years of unhealthy programming replacing it with a healthier, more motivated mindset. It allows the parts of us to become balanced so you can live the life that you have chosen.

The techniques utilised in this book are the same techniques utilised within the CaS Therapy Centre. The processes shared with you throughout this book have been developed through intense scrutiny, perfecting the program for people to embrace their new 'weigh of life'. The program empowers people to live the life they choose and become a shape and size that is right and healthy for them, part of which comes from giving up the struggle which is often attached to the sabotage part and can keep people stuck in the diet cycle. We will take you step by step through this process so you can begin to understand how the mind and body are connected. When you understand why that sabotage part comes into play, you will understand more about yourself when it comes to healthy eating and living. You can then begin to unravel the thought processes and uncover the actual core of the issue.

Stay with us as we review many advanced simple techniques that can help you arrive at where you want to go. This book is not about a 'diet'. It is about being healthy, living healthy, eating healthy, feeling healthy and thinking healthy and understanding the mind, the body and the parts of the mind; cleaning the slate, starting afresh, and establishing new, healthier habits and patterns of behaviour; approaching weight management in an easy and relaxed manner by simply adopting and embracing new and improved approaches; and seeing life through health-focused lenses, so life can begin to flourish and prosper.

Chapter 1
Living a Healthy Lifestyle – Weight Management – a Lifestyle Choice

We will guide you through how to create new patterns of behaviour and new thought processes by giving you the tools you need to control your cravings. By the time you complete this book, 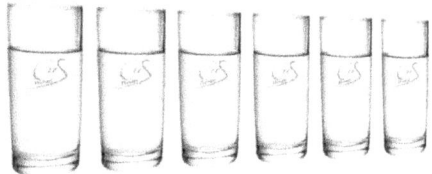 you will have many of the skills we share with our clients who partake in our weight management program, and the knowledge to recognise the body's parts and the signals they transmit. Plus you will know how to utilise the power of the mind to your advantage. You will discover the secrets of how to eat to refuel the body in a healthy manner, instead of eating as an emotional response to differing stimuli. You will be able to examine why you eat, the importance of good nutrition, and the benefits of water and the necessity of proper hydration.

> It is about making a clear and precise choice to be healthy, to live healthy, to eat healthy, to feel healthy and to think healthy and to convey a clear and precise message to the parts of the subconscious mind.

What is required is acceptance and acknowledgment. To realise that you deserve a healthy body and that you can have that healthy body. With the adoption of a different mental attitude, the process can really come down to it being a simple choice that involves making a clear and precise decision to be healthy, live healthy, eat healthy, feel healthy and think healthy, and conveying the clear and precise message to your subconscious mind.

You will notice that throughout the book one of the many focus points is about taking back your inner power and making the choices that you want to make, despite what, or who, stands in your way. Often we can continuously blame ourselves, or others, for the decisions we make when the decisions don't work out the way we may want, or we simply look at the world through the lenses that allow the voice to say, 'it is their fault.' 'It is the environment.' 'There wasn't anything else to eat.' 'He said that I was stupid,' or 'It was my friend who did it'. This language often leads to blaming others for our own actions, which does not allow the parts of you to grow and develop. Ostrow, a well-known Australian mind, body and soul writer, refers to blame as being disempowering, leading to a compulsion of repetition. Ostrow believed that 'taking responsibility empowers and allows you to alter your circumstance' (Ostrow, 2007, p. 111).

In society we are bombarded with conflicting messages regarding food. No wonder many of us struggle with weight issues. We spend millions of dollars on fad diets and diet products that never really address the core issues surrounding food and why we overeat.

If you truly believe that you will never be the shape and the size you want to be, then you are absolutely correct, you won't be. Beliefs can, and often do, hold people back from achieving what truly matters to themselves, as their beliefs have the ability to trample on everything and stop them from achieving their goals or desires. If you challenge that belief pattern and replace it with one that works, then you are on the right road for you to allow your body to be the vehicle that takes you through life in the direction that is right and healthy, a direction that is planned and coordinated. As you read on you will discover that this journey is one that you can travel on with ease and comfort if you choose and plan it to be that way.

Unfortunately, obesity is a worldwide health problem that brings major health risks, yet despite this we are still overeating and not participating in enough exercise. We believe that in order to understand why you overeat, or why you eat the way you do, you need to recognise why that part wants to keep the weight in the first place.

We have decided to share our knowledge so we can guide you to love and respect the body for the amazing, miraculous work of art that it is. With this appreciation for the body, you are likely not to overeat ever again. You will be able to confidently make choices that benefit the way you live, always striving for a healthy way of life. The word 'diet' has such a negative connotation. It does nothing to motivate you and constantly activates the deprivation part of you. When you think of the word 'diet', you may think of the struggle, the battle of the 'yoyo' diets and weight gain and weight loss. This, in turn, then continues to talk with the deprivation part of you, causing anguish and leaving space for any old behaviours that are not useful to return. The term 'healthy lifestyle' brings a very different image to mind. All of our internal parts have roles and are working with us and for us towards our best interests. However, these parts have different beliefs regarding what is in our best interests and can therefore be in conflict and in need of resolution. Most people think of increased energy and a lighter and brighter attitude when we think of a term like 'healthy lifestyle'. Living a life that is filled with choices, motivation and energy is within arm's reach.

Weight loss and language

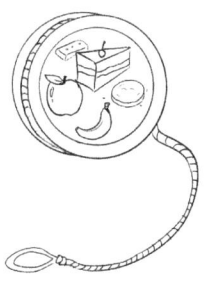

One of the most important things in weight management, living a healthy lifestyle and weight reduction is the concept of language. When you program in self-defeating language like 'I'm not good enough' or 'I cannot eat healthy' the mind holds on to that information and brings it into your reality. In order to change your thought processes you must first give the mind clear, clean, crisp and direct language because the subconscious mind does not analyse the information it gathers; it simply processes. You can think of the subconscious mind as an organic computer hard drive with your conscious mind being the random access memory or RAM.

The conscious mind filters the programming of your subconscious mind and the subconscious mind is solution focused. We like to use the analogy of losing your car keys as a good example. When you lose something, you turn the place upside down until you find whatever you have misplaced. When you lose something, you are also sending your subconscious mind a message that you must find it, thus the importance of setting the language scene now and forever.

What we usually do is tell ourselves that we want to lose weight; however, we do not actually want to lose weight, we actually want to throw it away. By saying 'losing' we are sending a message to the subconscious mind that we have lost something. As the subconscious mind is solution focused, it is receiving a message of a need to find what is lost. The truth is that your fat cells have memories, so when the fat drips away and the fat cells empty, the fat cells then have the inclination that they need to fill up with fat again.

Fat cells, also known as adipocytes, are like mini fuel tanks used to store energy for future usage (Medicine, 2007). Your fat cells also function as endocrine glands that secrete hormones and something called adipocytokines that communicate with your brain and other cells in the body.

A normal healthy adult body has about 25 to 30 billion fat cells! (Medicine, 2007). A typical overweight adult might have 75 billion fat cells. Adults who are severely obese can have up to 300 billion fat cells. An infant is born with about 5–6 billion fat cells and this number increases over childhood and throughout puberty. An overweight person's fat cells can be three times as large as a person with a normal body composition.

Research has shown that fat cells can multiply, however it usually only happens when there is a prolonged extensive weight gain. Research also tells us that fat cells have remarkable memories.

You are born with a certain number of fat cells. If you take in more calories than the body needs, your fat cells actually stretch to store the extra calories. You may in fact even gain more fat cells once your fat cells have engorged to their maximum size. The moment you create fat cells, they remain in the body forever. They may shrink as you drop in weight, however they seldom go away unless they are surgically removed.

Fat cells actually produce a variety of substances that have an influence on the body's weight. When you have enlarged fat cells or just too many fat cells, these substances are released into your bloodstream in higher levels than normal. The body becomes used to these higher levels and so do your fat cells, and this is one of the major reasons why you may find it difficult to drop the weight permanently.

Fat cells are not the only things that have extraordinary memories. Your subconscious mind also remembers very well. Heather recalls in her earlier 20s being a size 8–10, around 50 kg, and her perception of self was that she was still big in size. This is because as a child, she was ALWAYS told that she could never be anything else than big in size.

You need to be comfortable with the weight you are and be assertive to those who take it upon themselves to make comment. Often people place upon you their own values and beliefs about what they believe is right and healthy for you, and whilst it is not their place to judge what is right and healthy for you, you are unable to control what others may believe. However, what you can do is choose not to allow their intrusion. When you are born, you have the God given right, or whatever higher belief system you believe in, to control just one person and that one person is you and not another living soul on the planet.

For example, you may be very comfortable with the shape and size you are and others (often close friends or family members) take it upon themselves to make comment on your weight, thus attempting to alter your opinion of yourself so you may live by their values and beliefs. Some of the comments that we have both been personally subjected to include and are not limited to the following:

- 'You are going to grow up and be just like your grandmother, she was big too.'
- 'Oh, haven't seen you for a while, you have been in a good paddock.'
- 'Oh you are one of the short, barrel members of the family. When are you going to do something about that weight?'

These are obviously very hurtful comments and believe us when we say that the mind remembers these and every other hurtful comment people say to you over the years. This process you are about to undertake will change how you feel about yourself at a very deep level of the mind.

We love this quote by Marianne Williamson, an inspirational speaker and author, because it really portrays how we can think and feel about ourselves:

> Our deepest fear is not that we are inadequate. Our deepest fear is that we are powerful beyond measure. It is our light, not our darkness that most frightens us. We ask ourselves, 'Who am I to be brilliant, gorgeous, talented, fabulous?' Actually, who are you not to be? (Williamson).

The time has come to turn over a new leaf and feel better about yourself because you deserve it. If you have tried diets in the past, you might want to ask yourself if those diets were taking you in the right direction. If your answer is 'no', then you need to ask yourself if you are ready, willing and able to accept the consequences and live a healthier, more productive life as a result. When you ask the mind a 'yes' or 'no' question, there is no doubt as to the direction of the answer, because a 'yes' or 'no' question gives the mind clear, clean language.

Through the counselling process, which is filled with exploration, empowerment and the identification of useful and not so useful patterns and behaviours, your life can change the way you want it to and be reset into something that coincides with your values, beliefs and lifestyle. Resetting and reprogramming is only a matter of finding what works for you. Even when you utilise a process like hypnosis you are essentially reprogramming your subconscious mind from thoughts of disparity and struggle when it comes to weight loss, to thoughts of good health and vitality. You are essentially resetting your blueprint and your thought process when it comes to weight. As part of this process, you might discover that you were holding on to your weight for more than one reason. Sometimes we carry extra weight as a buffer or a

Chapter 1
Living a Healthy Lifestyle – Weight Management – a Lifestyle Choice

shield. Sometimes there is a payoff and the weight has actually served a purpose.

Everyone struggles with different issues when it comes to weight management and fitness. Some of us are addicted to sugar, while others are hung up on processed foods or fast foods. Whether or not you want to simply gain the motivation to exercise or gain the motivation to eat healthier, this book can help you shift your thinking so you are eating to live, rather than always living to eat.

Counselling, ego state therapy and hypnotherapy are such amazing and incredible ways to make changes in your life, because your thoughts create the world around you, every minute of every day, making them wonderful tools for weight management. We are so thrilled and elated that you have decided to take this journey with us because you deserve to be the best you can be.

Weight management and motivation

> This process you are about to undertake requires a shift in thinking, a lifestyle choice – the choice to be healthy.

If you have a desire to manage your weight and feel better, there is no better place to start than your motivation. Weight management is an emotional process. If you want to drop some weight and keep it off, you first have to understand the emotional connection that you have with food. You need to understand why you eat, why you overeat and what motivates you to do so.

The body is your temple and you only obtain one body per lifetime so it is important to treat it with the respect it deserves. Just like you would not put low grade or bad petrol into a fine sports car, you will also run more efficiently and effectively if you fuel the body with quality, healthy food that is right for your body.

In order for the weight to drip away and to keep it off, you have to first change the way you think and feel about food. You need to stop 'yoyo' dieting and trust in this process. You are the authority of your own mind, you can make this happen. Anything you want, you can do. Yes, really you can, providing it is physically possible and even then it may still not be impossible. Who would have ever thought man could run the four minute mile or fly to the moon. Yes, at some stage that was impossible in the minds of some and yet it was a dream and a goal within the minds of those who dared to challenge themselves and make the impossible possible.

This process you are about to undertake requires a shift in thinking, a lifestyle choice – the choice to be healthy. It's so simple – so easy. You can obtain optimum health and stay healthy by peacefully allowing the weight to drip away at a subconscious level.

The mind is so powerful, so strong. The mind creates your reality every second of every day. If you think you continually struggle with weight dripping away and eating healthy – then that is what will keep perpetuating in your life. If you change the way you think and feel about food on the inside – you can change the way you look and feel on the outside. Internal versus external will be further explored in our journey through the coming chapters.

How important is it to you for the weight to drip away? Obviously very important because you are reading this book. Now let us understand that we are all different, with unique strengths and different needs. The amount of weight to drip away can vary from 4 to 40 kilograms, or be any number. At the end of the day life is all about living a healthy lifestyle and allowing the weight to just continue to drip away. You will need to be kind to yourself and accept that you are responsible for you and that you are able to control you, if you choose. You will discover how to change your perspective and make the decision that you have had enough and that NOW is the time to 'do different', to change and live a healthy life. There are many different reasons why the weight is there and why we eat certain foods, when and who with, so discovering and understanding the true reasons behind your eating habits and associations can only direct you to the way of life you choose to live. We eat for many different reasons – for emotional comfort, for hunger, for good nutrition and even for things like relief from anger, anxiety or frustration.

Experts agree that up to 75% of overeating is actually caused by our emotions. We eat in response to our feelings instead of eating in response to our hunger.

Many of us grew up equating food with comfort and as a result we turn to food instead of looking to heal our emotions. Emotions can be uncomfortable, raw and painful and often difficult to manage.

Emotional eating becomes a natural habit over time which can cause us to eat when we are angry, frustrated, anxious, bored, lonely, stressed or a multitude of other emotions. The truth of the matter is that overeating does not do anything to comfort us emotionally – we just falsely believe it does.

The only thing overeating causes is extra weight gain, pain and anguish. By accepting and managing your emotions, you can discover and learn to substitute more appropriate techniques to work with your emotional issues. You can take food out of the equation and as a result feel better, think more clearly and look better.

> This process is a journey –
> a journey of discovery all about you.

Counselling, ego state therapy and hypnotherapy are processes that can help you change your subconscious thought patterns and behaviours – thought and behavioural patterns that have been with you perhaps for a very long time. If you struggle with weight issues, you know how important this is to you, you know now that there is an end to that struggle.

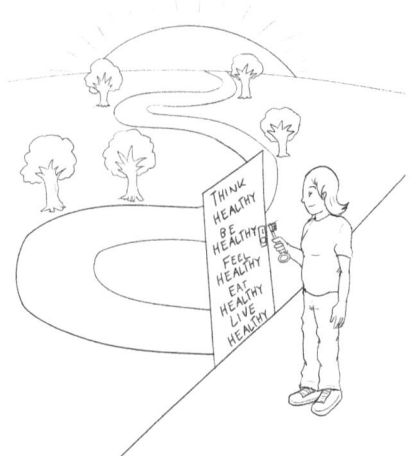

This process is a journey, a journey of discovery. This journey is an exploration of the inner spirit and of the soul. Discovering the reasons why you might sabotage yourself and the reasons why you are having difficulty managing weight and becoming healthy is life changing. This process is akin to a treasure hunt. As you read the following chapters, you will find many treasures along the way. Treasures that will help you turn that corner to improved health. Believe us when we say that you can have everything you want – vibrant health, increased energy and a happier and healthier lifestyle. However, in order to encompass these things, you need to first believe you are worthy and that you deserve the very best. From this moment onwards you only have the best and all you need to do is make a decision.

This book is much more than a simple book of exercises. It is about discovering the real you, the healthy you, the core essence of the internal and external self. This book incorporates the steps to remove layer upon layer so you can finally reveal your true essence and your true spirit. The chapters contain the content of dreaming up an enhanced lifestyle, and courageously walking the steps and pathway to be the best you can be for yourself. You will discover a core framework that will guide you to be the best you that you choose and live the best quality of life that is available to you.

> You do not have to stay trapped where you are; you can have the body and the vibrant health you are seeking and this is much easier than you might think.

Chapter 1
Living a Healthy Lifestyle – Weight Management – a Lifestyle Choice

There is a lot to cover on the road ahead, and we assure you that what you learn will be worth the journey. This process will really help you identify the origin of your weight issues.

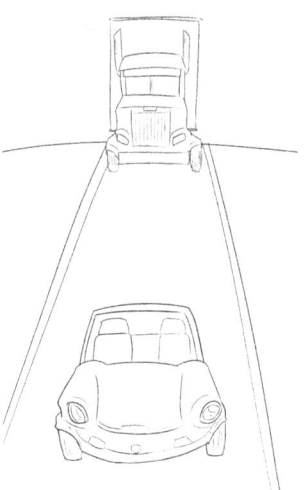

First and foremost, you need to recognise exactly where you are in this journey right now and make a firm decision where it is that you want to be. You may see yourself as a fully loaded, heavy truck which has difficulty manoeuvring around at the moment and you may wish to be more like a quick, slick, nimble well-kept sports car that performs very well.

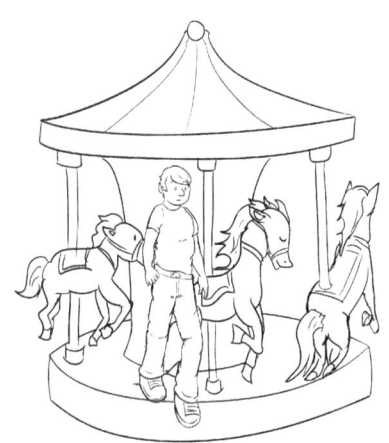

Before we start, let us look at some self-reflective questions that will help you become more aware of some of the most important issues you have, as you work through the chapters pertaining to weight management.

Now is the time to decide to make a change and set about jumping off the merry-go-round. Start a new and different lifestyle journey, a road of peace, calmness and balance. We are sure that you often feel like 'Here we go again' or maybe you have said to yourself 'I just have no willpower'. As we travel together on this journey, let us help you understand willpower, what it is and its role. Allow us to help and guide you to how you can choose to hop off this merry-go-round for good, just as easily as you are able to jump off the ride at the sideshow. Stop right now and make a decision to commit to yourself. Decide to 'do different', to change, to live differently, to release old habits and behaviours. This is happening right now and whilst you cannot change yesterday, you certainly can change today and alter the destinations of your tomorrows. The now is about deciding to take the steps you need to move you through the differing stages of change.

You do not need to formally do these in order for this process to be effective. These are just to create awareness around your particular issues regarding your weight. You can either jot down your answers in a journal or the NIB, or simply mull them over in the mind, however, writing it down makes it real.

Activity 1: Self-Reflective Questions

Self-reflective questions for weight management

1. Why do you really want to drop the weight? Be honest with yourself here.

2. What is your ultimate weight goal? What is the time frame you've allowed yourself to drop this weight? Is it realistic? If not, you can adjust it because this journey is not about deprivation; this process is about vibrant health.

3. Think about your weight management journey in terms of your highest weight and your lowest weight. Thinking about those times at your ideal weight or lowest weight, examine what was going on for you in your life at the time and take notes.

4. What kind of emotions do you equate with your weight when you think of your weight fluctuations? Were you especially happy and fulfilled when you were at your lowest weight or ideal weight? Were you stressed and anxious at your highest? Just think about how your emotions impacted on your weight.

5. Have you ever tracked what you are eating? There are many online tools and mobile phone apps that can help you do this.

Track your food consumption for a period of 2–3 days so you can honestly examine what you are eating. This is not about chastising yourself, it is about gaining self-awareness and noticing when you eat most. Emotional eating is a big one. (Emotional eating does not have to refer to a negative emotion; it can also be a happy emotion. Often we hear people say things like 'I am not emotional' and they've made that assumption because they do not cry. However, they overlook all of the other human emotions, such as being happy, glad, and angry.)

6. Examine the reasons you overeat and why? Are you eating to fulfil hunger or eating to bury emotions? You may not be aware why and that is okay.

7. Do you have a genetic predisposition to being overweight? If so, take heart, this can be changed! You do not have to continue the trend.

8. Do you ever use food as a reward? If so, why?

9. Are you using food to help overcome other problematic issues in your life? If so, this might be a good time to examine those.

10. Do you exercise on a regular basis or make time for walks? If not, can you make some time?

11. What do you believe is standing in your way of achieving and maintaining your healthy weight? Can you see yourself overcoming these obstacles? An important part is to be able to picture yourself at your ideal level of health, because change begins in the mind.

12. How willing are you to change? This process is life changing and if you are ready, willing and able, that is half the battle!

The most important aspect here is to embrace this process, which requires a commitment from YOU. This is not magic; therefore, the process does require a certain amount of commitment and dedication on your part. As you work through these exercises and chapters, you may discover some things about yourself that are hurtful or painful, and that is okay. This is a journey, not a destination. Remember the importance of being kind and gentle to yourself as you partake in this process. Nothing will change without changes from your end. If you are ready for the weight to drip away and to gain better health, then this journey will be a successful one. Our role is to assist you in this process and to help mediate and negotiate, and help you identify those obstacles and roadblocks that are keeping you from improved health. Let's not question everything; let's explore and learn.

So if you are ready, let's begin!

Chapter 2

Purpose – What is Behind Your Decision?

Examining what is behind your decision to manage your weight

To create new patterns of behaviour in order to heal and find the resolution needed, we need to first identify what the patterns are and what purpose they have served, including when they were developed in our childhood. This process promotes and allows the internal parts to reset and reevaluate what is right and healthy for you.

> It is not always about the weight; sometimes there are other reasons why you may hold on to excess weight.

Why do YOU want to drop the weight? Is your decision to undergo this process only about the weight, or are there other reasons?

We have discovered in our years of being therapists that it is not always about the weight. The weight is often a secondary issue to a much larger issue. If you have struggled for years with weight management in an effort to gain better health, examining what is behind your decision is of integral importance.

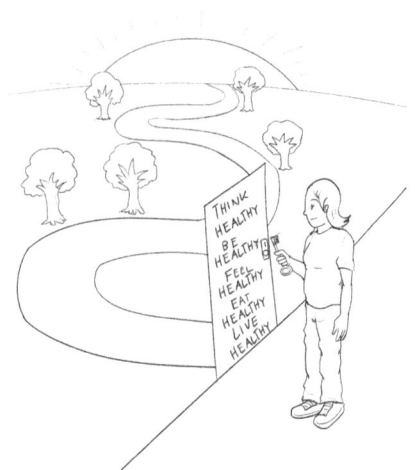

Just as this book is not about a 'diet', your decision to manage your weight is most likely not solely about the weight. The key is 'being healthy, living healthy, eating healthy, feeling healthy and thinking healthy'.

Think about your choices in terms of what is driving your decision to better manage your weight. Do you have the desire to live a healthier life? Do you have a yearning to feel better? How about a craving to have more energy, more motivation and more enthusiasm? What about your appearance? Know that it is okay if you merely just want to look better because confidence can go a long way to helping you live a better life.

Some people want to drop in weight to stave off chronic disease so they can age more gracefully. Obesity can lead to diabetes and heart disease and can be a contributing factor to other ailments such as kidney disease, hormonal imbalances and even cancer.

Sometimes your weight can keep you from living a well-balanced life. In other words, it holds you back. Perhaps you might decide to stay home instead of meeting friends for a walk. You might decide to stay in by yourself and watch a movie instead of meeting someone for dinner because you may subconsciously feel intimidated about people watching you eat. Being unhappy with your weight and not feeling at home in the body can even keep you from establishing and maintaining healthy relationships, because subconsciously you may avoid people and places.

Think about the reasons you make certain choices. Why do you do some of the things you do? The fact that you are here continuing to read our message means that you are serious about this process. You are willing

Chapter 2
Purpose – What is Behind Your Decision?

to make a commitment to yourself. You can be very proud of yourself already for how far you have come.

> Achieving and maintaining a healthy weight is
> not about a diet – it is about a lifestyle.

Making this commitment and taking stock of where you are is an important first step in your weight management journey. Committing to action is something that you are in control of and have a choice of whether you do or you do not. Discovering what is behind the decision to do different and what is behind the choices you make can go a long way to helping you achieve your goals.

When you make the choice to pursue a healthier lifestyle you take on a new mental attitude. You begin to realise that weight management is really a very simple process. With the right mental attitude change becomes much easier to accept and becomes an everyday part of life.

We need to have the conscious mind and the subconscious mind working together as a team. Sometimes one might start a weight management program and be doing really well and then all of a sudden stop making progress. What happens is you begin reverting back to your old habits because the subconscious mind is used to the old habits and behaviours and it takes time for new habits and behaviours to form.

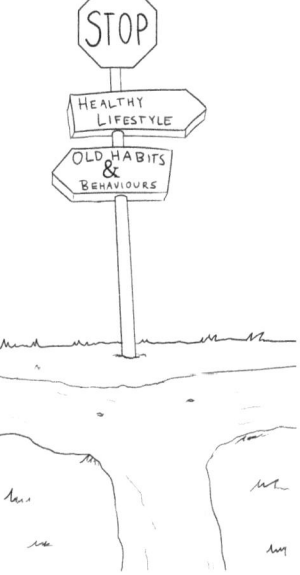

You may discover that an old belief system is taking over because of what you are telling yourself subconsciously. You may be telling yourself in the mind: 'Every time I have done this before I go down to a certain weight and I just cannot do it anymore' or 'I don't know what it is that stops me'.

Well, there is your answer! You are telling yourself, 'I go to this weight and I stop, I give up, I throw in the towel', so that is what you are programming yourself and the subconscious to believe is true. The key is to validate that unhelpful talk and to control that thinking. When a thought like that does enter the mind (and it will), simply acknowledge it, thank it for the message and continue saying to yourself: 'I am now living a healthy lifestyle and I always will. I deserve to look, feel and be healthy.'

> The theory behind change is all about altering those mental thought processes. When you begin repeating healthy positive thoughts, the mind begins to move in a healthy positive direction.

When you hear or read a suggestion, you really need to adopt one of four mental attitudes at the conscious level. What mental attitude you do adopt at the conscious level allows that suggestion to enter your subconscious mind, and when you do allow it into your subconscious mind that is when real change actually begins.

If you reject a suggestion, there will be no change and, unfortunately, that is one mental attitude you could and do sometimes choose. Explore how often this might occur and listen to your findings. Observe that you are noticing your thoughts, feelings and actions.

> Mindfulness is a mental state of awareness, openness and focus. When we are mindful, we are able to engage fully in what we are doing, let go of unhelpful thoughts and act effectively without being pushed around by your emotions (Harris R., 2010, p. 5).

If you reject a healthy suggestion, it could be that the suggestion sounds a little bit uncomfortable to you for some particular reason and if that is the case, the suggestion will automatically be rejected and not be allowed into the subconscious mind.

Another possibility could be that you are just a little bit blasé about the suggestion and you do not really care too much about it, therefore, you are not passionate about it. Again, change will not happen. You are in control of the choices you have in front of you. You will soon be able to steer towards helpful and useful choices that create the pathway you have chosen. Remember, if you want change to occur, you need to '**commit to action**' and let the vehicle drive to where you choose to go.

The other mental attitude you could adopt, which is most dangerous and very common when people give up, is that when you hear the suggestion, you like the idea of the suggestion and *hope* it works. The words 'hope' and 'try' need to be eliminated from your vocabulary, when you are referring to yourself. It is okay to 'hope' for someone else, however when it comes to your destiny you need to 'plan', not 'hope.' In the next chapter we look and explore the meanings of the words 'hope' and 'try' in relation to the subconscious mind and why they need to be eliminated extensively.

You might be asking at this point why words like 'hope' and 'try' would have a negative connotation. We will speak more about this later, however the words 'hope' and 'try' basically set you up for failure. For example, if you say 'I will try and make it', a part of you is saying you have no intention of making it. The word 'hope' has the same kind of unhelpful connotation. If you say something like 'I hope I can win that scholarship', there is still a part of the mind that is clinging to the idea that you will NOT win the scholarship. 'Hope' is not a very strong word of commitment to say to oneself.

If you are *trying* to manage your weight – that is non-committal; you are either committed to dropping weight or you are not.

Much of this is about semantics – you drank the water or you did not. Even if you drank a little bit, you still drank something, so it is 'yes' or 'no', not a 'try'. There is no grey area here. The truth is that black and white and crisp, clear, clean language works and is accepted into the subconscious mind much better than language that is non-committal.

Here are some other examples. You are either pregnant or you are not. You are not a little bit pregnant! You don't 'try' and cross the road. You either cross the road or you do not cross the road. Even if you are walking very slowly, placing one foot in front of the other, you are still actually 'doing' the action of crossing the road.

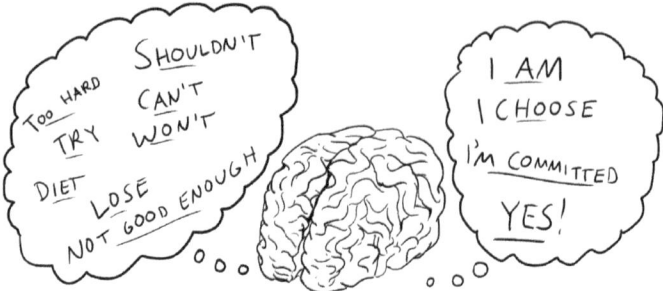

When you make a firm, positive decision to change and you make that commitment to 'be healthy, live healthy, eat healthy, feel healthy and think healthy' you provide the mind with clear, concise language that is easy to follow. This kind of positive mental attitude can help you make some amazing changes in your life.

As we have mentioned, parts of the mind can be in conflict. One may say 'I'm not good enough' whilst another part says 'Yes, I am committed'. Often these parts can become conflicted, impacting on thoughts and behaviours. These parts need to have conflict resolution so they can help you move forward.

According to Dr Russ Harris (2007), author of *The Happiness Trap*, it is easy to become caught up in comparing yourself to others. The mind might dredge up unpleasant memories from the past, find fault with your life or even drag you into scary scenarios about the future about things that might go wrong. Dr Harris specialises in Acceptance & Commitment Therapy (ACT), which speculates that the root of all suffering lies within the human language itself, as opposed to the mind (Harris R. , 2007). On a positive note, language helps us form maps and models of the world, which helps us relate to other people. On a less positive note, we might also use language to lie, deceive, manipulate or incite hatred. The

Chapter 2
Purpose – What is Behind Your Decision?

premise behind ACT is that it helps 'to create a rich, full and meaningful life while accepting the pain that inevitably goes with it' (Harris R., 2009, p. 7). Living life is about **'*experiencing the experiences*'** which leads to living a life that has difference within its emotions, thoughts and feelings. As human beings, experiencing feelings and emotions is what makes us unique to our species, **'*feeling the feeling*'** in our moments of life.

Dr Harris also says that thanks to the human language the mind can conjure up pain at any moment. The mind can also cause us to become caught up in unfavourable comparisons or negative self-judgments such as 'I am too fat' or 'I am not smart enough' or 'I am not pretty enough'. The mind might also cause us to focus too much on those painful memories, even on our happiest days. When you learn how to manage and make room for those painful thoughts and feelings, you can begin to live a rich, meaningful life, one that matters to you. All thoughts and feelings are a part of our everyday life and influence what we think and do, enhancing our experiences. If we did not go through those painful thoughts and hurtful feelings that everyone encounters throughout their life, we would simply be existing and not living a life that is full of purpose and different experiences. It is about making room, creating space for all thoughts and feelings, as this is what makes us stand out from the rest. Actually, it's what makes us human. By making room specifically for painful thoughts and feelings, we can remove the power that those thoughts and feelings carry, perhaps forcing us to say and do things that we don't want to do. An example would be if you saw a cat become hurt by a car and the cat perhaps died. Most would become emotional as this is a sad experience. Our thoughts might be manifested into memories of past deaths or experiences with animals. Whatever the case, there may have been a trigger that brought on that emotion to the stimulus of the cat dying. If we did not have the ability to experience those feelings that were attached to those thoughts, you could simply say 'Oh, the cat died, let's go shopping', therefore having no real emotion. When we do not experience the feeling or emotion we simply become robotic to our stimulus which means we are disconnecting and not engaging in the world. Human emotions include having the experiences of being shocked, upset, angry or sad as these emotions can be attached to thoughts, thus the reason it is important to accept the grieving of losing a cat. Feeling is all about being part of what makes us human.

ACT uses six core therapeutic processes which can help you process painful and hurtful thoughts and emotions:

1. Contacting and connecting to the present moment, learning to be in the here and now, meaning to actually be here, in the here and now.
2. Defusion, observing your thinking and having choices around what you do with your thinking.
3. Acceptance or opening up, making room within us.
4. Looking at the self-as-context or pure awareness.
5. Having values or knowing what matters.
6. Committed to action or doing what it takes to live the life that you choose according to your values and not just your feelings.

While this book is not necessarily promoting ACT, the premise behind it is sound. ACT breaks mindfulness skills into three categories:

1. Defusion: distancing from, and letting go of, unhelpful thoughts, beliefs and memories.
2. Acceptance: making room for painful feelings, urges and sensations, and allowing them to come and go without struggle.
3. Contact with the present moment: engaging fully with your here-and-now experience, with an attitude of openness and curiosity (Harris R. , 2007).

Much like Dr Harris' model, we would like to assist you so that you can learn to accept and acknowledge the mind's thoughts and feelings while not being constantly driven by them every moment of every day. By accepting that you have unhelpful thoughts and gently acknowledging them, you can process those thoughts, move beyond and learn to replace them with more helpful thoughts and feelings. The following chapters contain many strategies to help you connect to self and others and accept and make room for your thoughts and feelings, exploring values and beliefs that resonate with you and techniques to help you **commit to action** to change your life permanently. All you need to do is make that decision to 'do different'.

> The good news is that, although we can't avoid such pain, we can learn to handle it much better – to make room for it, rise above it and create a life worth living (Harris R., 2007).

Discovering your purpose in life – what drives you?

People need to have a purpose in life. This is all about having a purpose with your choices. It is important to ask yourself the question, 'Do I want to live a healthy lifestyle?' If you live a healthy lifestyle, most likely you will achieve your purpose much easier than if you are not living a healthy lifestyle. Now, you may be able to survive and exist without living a healthy lifestyle, however the fact remains, if you are not healthy, you may have trouble achieving certain goals or living the quality of life you choose because your health or your weight may actually be holding you back.

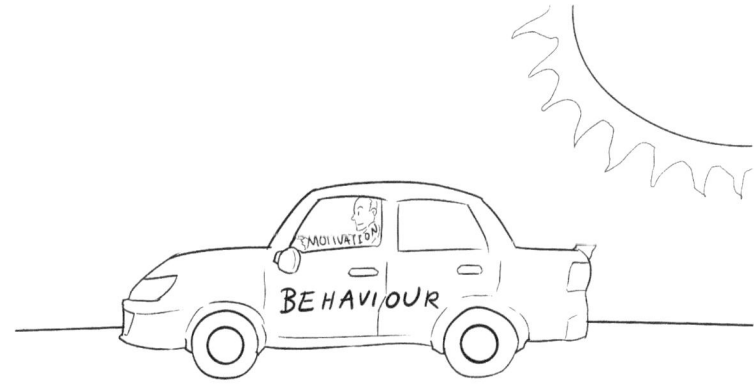

Ask yourself now – is your weight holding you back? It is alright to admit this, because the fact is you have already come a long way on this journey and as you continue to read on, you are already displaying that you are committed to this process.

> The simple fact is that it is not always about the weight – there is so much more to weight.

You may have heard this many times before; however, it is worth repeating. In order to achieve a goal or desire for something, you need to straighten out and organise your head first. Preparation is 'the key'. The brain needs to have a focus point and you need to be prepared, whether your goal is managing your weight or finishing an important project.

This is true with weight management or any other goal you may strive for in your life. When you first say you are going to go on a diet you are leaving everything up to your willpower and willpower lives in the conscious mind. In order for true change to occur, you need to change the programming of the subconscious mind, just like a computer hard drive. It is all about '**Choice Power**'. We have discovered that in order to execute your choices you need power to do so. It's all about internal control. We have developed a method to power those choices which we like to call '**Choice Power**'. **Choice Power** has a stronger drive both consciously and subconsciously. **Choice Power** will be the stronger road to take to help you move forward. **Choice Power** allows you to action the commitment to do different and live the life you choose. We will always gain more if we choose to not always do what is easiest, rather, what is best. We have known many who have adopted the philosophy 'Do what is best, not what is easiest' and how this had helped change their way of thinking and doing, bringing about a better lifestyle filled with informed choices. Wanting to do what is best is similar to wanting to see the greatest scenic view. You almost always have to take the uphill road requiring more energy, however the benefits and the results are worth the experience, one to remember and reflect upon.

Chapter 2
Purpose – What is Behind Your Decision?

So what happens is you decide that you are feeling uncomfortable with your weight. You then decide that you wish to 'lose' some weight. Your willpower kicks in and you focus, doing everything correctly to achieve your goal weight or at least arrive at a more comfortable place.

Your willpower is then satisfied it has reached the goal weight or a place where it is comfortable and it relaxes. At that point the programming within the subconscious mind kicks in and as the subconscious mind is solution focused, it says: 'I've lost something and I must find it'. Then it usually does. It finds all that weight it has 'lost' and often a little bit more, hence the yoyo diet. We are sure you agree this is not a cycle you want to consciously keep repeating.

This is NOT a diet, this is a weigh (way) of life. So from this point on, we ask you to open your mind to be thinking and feeling that you are 'now living a healthy lifestyle and you always will'. To be effective and affirmative, the decision needs to be firmly made to live, be, feel, eat and think healthy.

We aim to help you discover how you can make different choices; choices that help the body thrive and not merely survive. Let's welcome '**Choice Power**' into our lives, because choices are made every single moment of every day. **Choice Power** can only empower you to be the person you choose to be, NOW.

As Bill Harris (2002) refers to as his 9 Principles for Happiness and Healing, we create our experience of life and can create the experience we want. In order to do this, the conscious awareness needs to be heightened, noticing those automatic thoughts and behaviours, making the conscious decision to change and bring forth the new thoughts and behaviours. There is one important element to all of this; you need to know that YOU have the power to change and to have the experiences that you choose to have. The first step is to make that decision.

The following process will assist you in moving forward, commit to change and embrace growth.

Harris' 9 Principles, which are very similar to the CaS Therapy's 7 Core Principles, demonstrate that the mind requires a sequence to ensure structural change for permanency.

1. Let whatever happens be okay.
2. Threshold.
3. Chaos and reorganization.
4. The map is not the territory.
5. Responsibility as empowerment.
6. Conscious change.
7. Witnessing.
8. Good and bad generalizations.
9. The neutral universe (Harris B. , 2002, p. 119).

The CaS Therapy 7 Core Principles focus on conscious awareness and letting go of anything that serves no purpose for you to move forward on your chosen pathway.

The CaS Therapy 7 Core Principles are based on conscious and subconscious stages to bring about change and growth, both within the conscious and subconscious states.

There are seven core principles that once understood, implemented and practised can lead you to master the direction in which you drive your life. Each principle may take some transitional time as you adjust your lifestyle. Remember, for all the changes and the growth to take place, validate and make room for those thoughts and feelings if and when the road becomes uncomfortable for a short period of time before permanent change takes place.

The Five Stages of CaS (Conscious and Subconscious) Therapy are:

- **Stage One**: Subconscious and not competent.
  Both the conscious and the subconscious have no knowledge and no skill.
  E.g. When you are first learning to drive a car.

- **Stage Two**: Conscious and not competent.
  The conscious gains knowledge, yet is still learning.
  E.g. You now know what is required to drive, however you do not have the practical experience.

- **Stage Three**: Conscious and competent.
  The conscious now has the knowledge and the ability to apply this knowledge.
  E.g. You now have the skills to drive the car with concentration.

- **Stage Four**: Subconscious and competent.
  The process is becoming easier through repetition.
  E.g. To drive a car now seems to be an automatic process.

- **Stage Five**: Conscious and Subconscious, Competent and Skilled.
  With constant repetition all four elements above have formed a strong automatic working relationship.
  E.g. After several years the task of driving a car is second nature and a process that requires no conscious focus or effort.

Each stage transitions into the next, strengthening the skill of the behaviour, and then they all integrate into the 7 Core Principles of the CaS Therapy framework.

Once mastered, you have a secure and permanently built pathway to smoothly, travel on – living the healthy lifestyle that you have planned and chosen to live.

The CaS Therapy 7 Core Principles

The activities throughout the book are based on the CaS Therapy 7 Core Principles. These principles are as follows:

1. Foundation – Discovery of where and how the beliefs were originally formed.

2. Language – Consciously relaying the language to the subconscious mind.

3. Growth – Planting the seeds.

4. Release – Cleaning the slate.

5. Reprogramming – Imprinting.

6. Connecting – Resetting the internal dialogue systems.

7. Preservation – Monitoring and maintaining.

Each of the seven principles have been thoroughly worked through to ensure that the principles work effectively and easily to incorporate change, both consciously and subconsciously. When Cas identified and explored her foundations of life at the time, in order to establish a new foundation, she found that experiencing different and challenging emotions such as hurt, anger, sadness and confusion brought new lenses to her view and perception of the world. Her belief began to change when she understood that even though the developmental years had been influenced by your parents, you can change your belief system if you strongly trust your own values. We often blame our parents for our behaviours: 'Never had enough love', 'never enough food', 'never was good enough' or 'I did things the way my parents wanted them to be, this is why I am the way I am'. When do you as an adult take charge and own your responsibilities and remove the restraints that you have placed around yourself to live the life you want to live and not the life that your parents wanted for you? This is your life and you won it despite what you think. Now is the time to want it, so take hold and commit to action.

Reasons you may hold on to weight subconsciously – secondary gains

A secondary gain is an indirect benefit. For example, there is a theory that people might choose to hold on to excess weight so they do not have to deal with the attention that a slim, healthy physique might bring them. Another example might be a child who fakes a sickness or a minor illness to draw extra attention. Now, we are not saying that you are holding on to excess weight on purpose. What we are saying is that there may be parts within the subconscious mind that may choose to hold on to the extra weight. Those parts are likely to hold the belief that the reason why they hold this weight is beneficial and positive for you.

There are many reasons why you may choose, consciously or subconsciously, to hold on to excess weight. Let's look at a few here.

- You want to stay inside your protective 'shield'.
- You do not like being the centre of attention.
- Your weight makes you feel 'safe'.
- You do not want to become obsessed with weight management.
- You like your 'comfortable' clothes.
- You are tired of 'dieting'.
- You want to be 'strong' not skinny.
- You actually like your body just like it is.
- You are afraid to fail.
- You are afraid to confront painful emotions.
- You have suffered from trauma and/or abuse.
- You love to eat.

- You do not want to deprive yourself.
- You like feeling comfortable surrounded by extra weight.

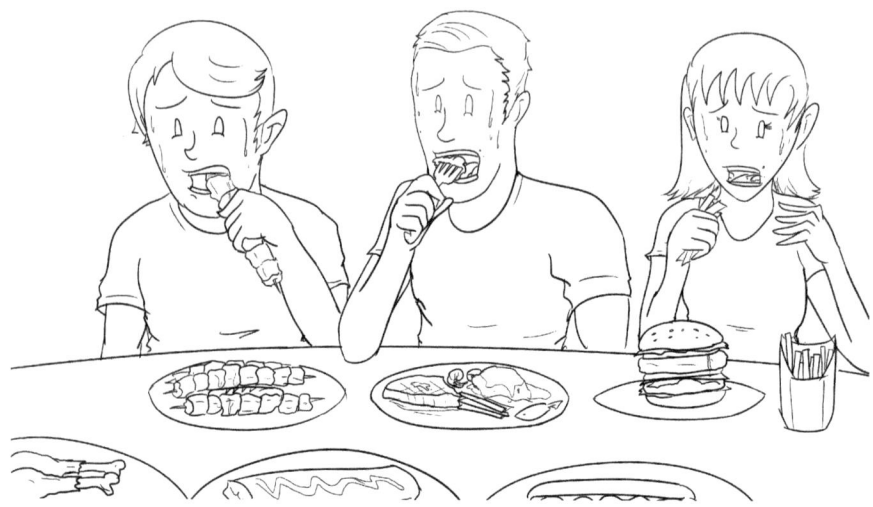

Do any of these sound familiar?

Hopefully you now understand the premise behind a secondary gain. Before we move on, take a moment to contemplate some of the reasons why you might subconsciously choose to hold on to extra weight. Take your time, even come back to this later if you choose. Be as honest as you can with yourself, as this is your life and how you want to 'do different' begins with 'YOU'. Remember to use the NIB.

Chapter 2
Purpose – What is Behind Your Decision?

ACTIVITY 2: REASONS
Reasons why I may *subconsciously choose* to hold on to excess weight:

1. _____

2. _____

3. _____

4. _____

5. _____

6. _____

7. _____

8. _____

9. _____

10. _____

Listing those reasons why you want to do things differently now!

ACTIVITY 3: REASONS TO DO DIFFERENT

Everyone needs a purpose in life. Everyone needs a reason to be. If you have no purpose, life can be pretty dull. It may sound great to be on a permanent 'vacation', however, a little goes a long way. We all need a purpose so we need to know, 'Why is it I am here?'

This process is all about making different decisions, healthier choices. It is about taking a new road, the road to better health. It is about making the definitive choice to 'do different' from this point forward. It is about making that commitment to change. When you have a purpose in life, you have a target, something to strive towards, a reason to be. When you can identify your 'purpose', you can make better, more informed decisions.

ACTIVITY 4: MY LIFE PURPOSE

What is your purpose?

What is that one thing you do that makes you shine?

What is that thing that everyone is always saying you are great at?

Think about this now and ask the mind to reveal to you what your life purpose is and contemplate this for a while.

Why do you climb out of bed each day?

What is it that makes you, YOU?

Chapter 2
Purpose – What is Behind Your Decision?

My life purpose

1. What do I want?
   _____

2. What is my purpose in life?
   _____

3. What is my reason to be?
   _____

Let's look at some other questions you can ask yourself to help you identify your life purpose:

1. What do you LOVE to do?
2. What is it you ALWAYS notice?
3. What would you do for FREE?
4. What do you love to LEARN about?
5. What do you love to TALK about?
6. What would you REGRET never doing?
7. If someone were able to look in your library, what would they find?
8. What SPARKS your creativity?
9. If you had all of the money you wanted and needed, and did not 'have to work', what would you do with your time?

Simply ask the mind to reveal to you now what your true purpose is and write down ANYTHING that comes to mind. This can be a word, a phrase, a sentence or even a picture or a symbol. Repeat this exercise until you write an answer that brings forth emotion. Take some time to create the space, to allow the subconscious mind to answer truthfully.

The answer that shall be revealed will be your life's purpose and you will recognise it instantly for the emotion will come forth.

ACTIVITY 5: EXERCISE TO REVEAL LIFE PURPOSE

Clear the mind of all the clutter. Begin by taking a deep breath in and out. Allow the mind to quiet. Just relax the mind and the body by continuing to breathe gently. You might even imagine you are breathing in a beautiful soft colour and this colour is gently loosening any strain or tension. As you continue to breathe deeply, feel this wonderful relaxation travelling down throughout the body.

The breath is so calming and healing, just allow your breath to quiet the mind. Observe the breath as it moves into and around the body. You may continue this deep breathing until you feel a sense of supreme relaxation. You may even imagine the body just melting away stress and tension.

Trust your intuition and go with the first thing that comes to mind. You can also grab a clean white sheet of paper and a pen or pencil and complete this exercise.

After the mind becomes clear and centred, ask yourself what your life purpose is.

Note anything that 'enters' into the mind.

You may see pictures in your mind or you may just receive impressions. Whatever you see is fine because everything has meaning.

Chapter 2
Purpose – What is Behind Your Decision?

Now ask yourself in this very calm, serene state of mind what you can do today to start moving towards this life purpose. What kind of decisions can you make to bring you closer to this goal?

Now ask yourself in this relaxed state of mind if your life would be easier if you were healthy and vibrant? Would it be easier for you to fulfil your purpose? There is no time like the present to begin making changes in your life. The fact is you can start TODAY. You can choose to live a healthier life, beginning right now. The choice is yours to make, you make choices all day, every day, starting the moment you wake up with the choice to 'rise and shine' or 'snuggle and cuddle', and so the choices continue throughout your day.

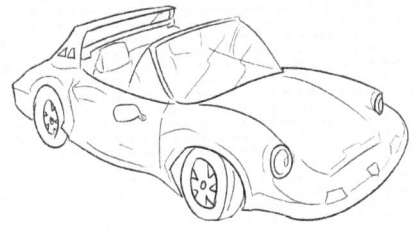
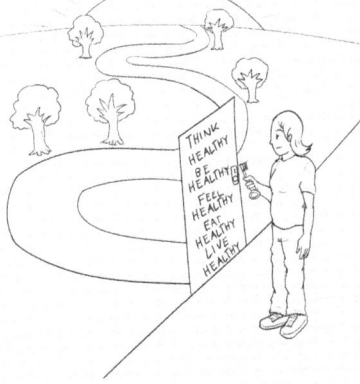

Take a moment to imagine how wonderful life is now that you are in this new vibrant state of health. Picture yourself creating better choices and making improved decisions. Notice how much easier life is when you are healthy and vibrant. Remember the car analogy, your body is your vehicle, the vehicle needs direction, nurturing and love, you have the choice to choose what vehicle you want to drive. This is about you taking back control and living your life, the life you want!

What type of car would you choose?

> What colour do you want your car to be and where do you want to drive to?
>
> Now imagine driving in the direction you choose, filled with creative choices and nurturing the body, in the vehicle you have chosen.
>
> How does that feel? What do you notice? Note it in the NIB.

You may repeat this exercise as many times as you desire. Remember, whatever the mind creates, the mind can heal and change. The mind is a very powerful tool and you can use the mind to make any changes you desire.

Chapter 3

'Try' and 'Hope'

What is your relationship with food?

> The process of weight management is not about
> deprivation and loss; it is about respect – respecting
> the food and respecting the body.

Do you have a love–hate relationship with food? You may have if you are struggling to throw away weight. It is important to note that food is not the enemy; it is also not the answer, a substitute, or a solution to dealing with emotions.

Food is fuel for the body, like petrol is fuel for the car, helping and giving you strength, clarity and the ability to maintain energy. Without the right kind of petrol, the car will not run efficiently. This is about you eating differently and changing your relationship with food. The process of weight management is not about deprivation; it is about respect; respecting yourself, respecting the body and respecting food, learning to work with those parts of the mind and gaining internal control. The process is more about your perception and your interpretation of language coupled with your relationship with food and how you digest your own experiences whilst living and engaging in the world.

When you remove words like TRY and HOPE from your vocabulary, you take on a new mental attitude. As we suggested in the previous chapter, the words 'try' and 'hope' are not strong words because they are non-committal and are words that are confusing to the subconscious mind.

If you say 'I will try and eat healthier' or 'I hope I can learn to eat healthier' you are suggesting to the subconscious mind that a part of you is not truly committed to eating healthier.

For example, if your friend invites you for dinner and you really do not want to go, some people will find themselves saying something like, 'I will *try* and be there, I will see how I go as I have to wait for a phone call.' What this really means is, 'I would rather not, but I don't want to hurt your feelings by telling you up front that I don't wish to go, so I will say I will try and justify why I didn't turn up after the event.' Sound familiar? Whereas, if you really wanted to go, you would say something like, 'Sure! What time do we need to be there? Do you want me to bring anything? Great, I'll see you there.' See the difference in the responses? The second one is a firm commitment with the clear intention that you certainly plan to attend.

The point is that if you were truly committed to something, you would walk on hot coals to make it happen. You would find a way, no matter what the circumstances. You do what matters.

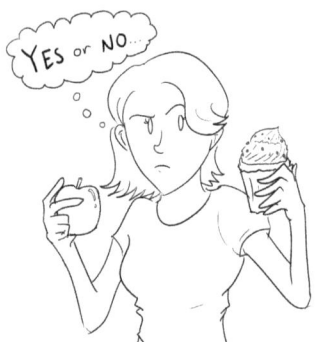

This development is really about self-discovery and learning to be more comfortable with yourself, your body and your decisions. It is 'okay' to feel 'not okay', to feel uncomfortable before you become comfortable. As you throw away the weight and allow the weight to drip away it is important to feel comfortable. When you do not feel comfortable in the body, you may have a tendency to wear clothing that is a little too big. In other words, you may not wear clothes that fit tightly or snugly to the body.

Chapter 3
'Try' and 'Hope'

When the weight begins to drop away, you can make a firm commitment to this process by throwing away your old oversized clothing. We suggest you begin to wear clothing that fits firmly on the body. Put on a belt and begin to feel the body and become comfortable in a smaller body. You can wear smaller sized skivvies and learn to feel more comfortable in clothing that hugs the body. Allow the body to transition into its new shape and size, the shape and size that is right and healthy for you. How your mind filters, perceives and interrupts that message whilst wearing the belt is the significant change that is desired in order to move forward.

It is important not to fold up those oversized items of clothing and put them back in the wardrobe, as the message you are sending to the subconscious mind is that you are only 'trying' and this is not a permanent lifestyle change, because you are keeping those clothes for when you become a big size again. By throwing them out of your wardrobe, you are giving the subconscious mind a clear message that you intend for this change to be permanent.

> Food does not have to be the enemy; food can be an enjoyable experience. Food fuels my body and keeps me functioning.

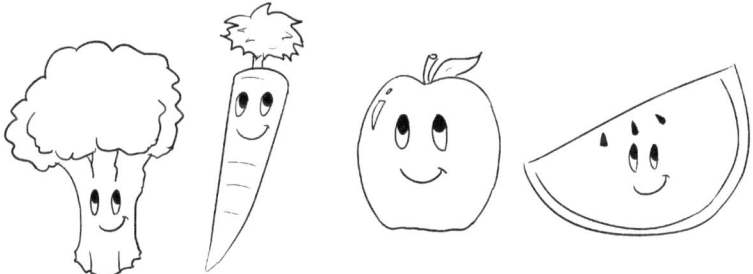

You can still enjoy food. We are not here to take that away from you. Quite the contrary, you can choose to eat foods that support a healthy body and a healthy lifestyle. Sometimes it is hard to appreciate food when you are living a hectic and frantic lifestyle. Eating on the run is not conducive to a healthy lifestyle, however, you can change this if you

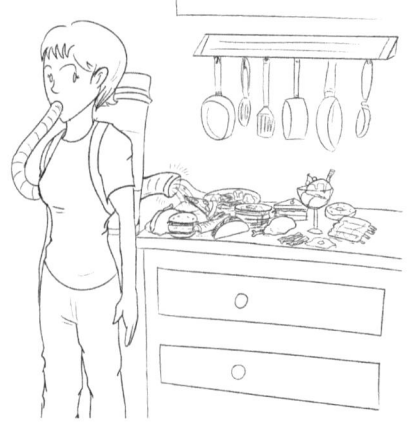

choose. Many people in today's busy society often inhale their food like a vacuum cleaner as they walk past the kitchen or eat while working at their desk. When you begin to practise mindful eating, you change your relationship with food. When you eat food more slowly and take time to appreciate the flavours, the colours and textures, you begin to value and enjoy food more. You seek out foods that nourish the body instead of merely filling the body.

When you eat mindfully, you gain real awareness and a connection between the mind and the body. You begin to appreciate food much more and you may even discover that you do not mind leaving food on the plate (refer to chapter 7 on Old Beliefs and Patterns for further information). Take a moment to notice what your mind is telling you now, then note it in the NIB. Reflecting is a powerful way to really bring that awareness around your relationship with food. Raising your awareness specifically around food can bring about the change that you want to occur. Having awareness is half the fun of learning and growing; the other half is full of choices and experiences.

Feeding the mouth and the mind

Often we experience feelings that cause **emotional responses** which result in eating all the wrong foods and far too much of them at any given sitting. We simply feed the mouth and the mind in an automatic action which becomes a slave to the body in a way that results in undesired behaviours.

Now is the time to take back control and feed the mouth in a way that is healthy and right for you. All you need to do is simply be mindful

Chapter 3
'Try' and 'Hope'

of what, when, where and how you are eating. All are very important elements to take back your self-power.

- Feeding the mouth takes practise before it becomes automatic.
- When you have satisfied your stomach the most important action to take now is to satisfy the mind and the mouth.

ACTIVITY 6: FEEDING THE MOUTH AND THE MIND

Make a list of whatever you think will help keep your mind and mouth busy in a healthier and happier way. Note it in the NIB.

For example: If you need to eat some chocolate because those cravings are completely out of control, break off one small piece of the block. Place the piece on the roof of the mouth and suck the chocolate until it dissolves completely. Then 5 minutes after eating the chocolate have a cold drink.

Remember, we only taste for approximately 2 minutes. After those 2 minutes have lapsed we no longer taste. The tastebuds have done their job; they have told you what that taste was, and then they go back to sleep, ready to be awaken for their next job. We are eating just for the simple reason that it is there, not because you love the taste. Really! Yes really, we think that we must eat more to taste that taste. Tasting is all in the way that you design yourself to think, wait, then wait again, then taste and articulate that taste like the activity took you through.

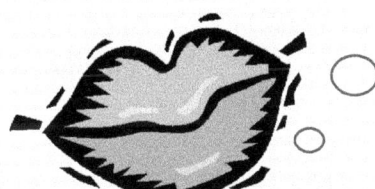

What do I taste?
What do I smell?
What do I hear?
Is it rough or smooth?
How is my body responding?

How motivated are you to drop weight and gain better health?

How motivated are you when it comes to dropping the weight and gaining better health? There are many reasons why we eat. If you find you are an impulsive eater and you eat for reasons other than hunger, you may need to dig a little deeper to discover why you feel the way you feel. The truth of the matter is that food does not offer you emotional comfort, no matter what you think. Food cannot fill an emotional void and you cannot fill your empty heart via your stomach, even if you think you can. If you are an impulsive eater, there may be other areas in your life causing you to overeat that you need to look at.

Being committed to this process and being committed to gaining better health will assist you in discovering reasons why you may tend to reach for food, and this commitment may lead you to seek life changing emotional support. The reality is that you need food to survive and thrive. When you commit to this healthy lifestyle process you are making a commitment to yourself, for better health, both on an emotional and physical level.

Why you eat – uncovering unhealthy associations

Think for a moment about a baby. A baby has the ideal weight management system. A baby cries when the baby is hungry and most likely stops eating when satisfied. Most infants do not eat any more than they need to eat, and if by chance they do eat more than they really need, they vomit it up, letting the parent know they have already had all that they need to eat. Therefore a baby's feeding system is the ideal blueprint for weight management that we have learnt and chosen to ignore over time.

In essence, this is the system that we want to adopt once more. We want to head back to that comfortable mollified blueprint and weight management system we had as a child. As a small child, usually we immediately stopped eating when we received the message and noticed the signal that we felt satisfied.

> When you begin to tune in to the body, you start to notice those feelings, signals and messages that the stomach is sending you; you begin to notice what you are noticing.

You may receive messages or notice the feelings that you are hungry and empty. Begin by acknowledging that it is okay to be hungry. In fact, it is okay to be hungry three times per day: just before breakfast, just before lunch and just before dinner. If you feel hungry and empty at other times, you can ask the body what else it may need besides food. First, ask yourself, where are you really hungry? Is it in the mind or the stomach? Check first to see if you are thirsty, as those signals of feeling hungry and feeling thirsty are close cousins and feel similar.

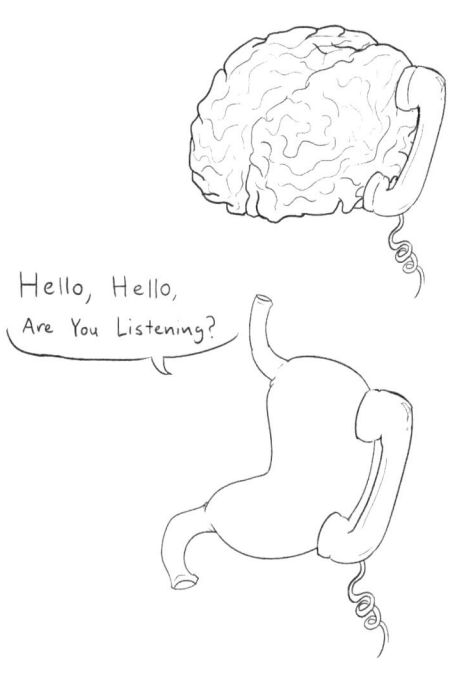

You can then tune in to the body when you start to eat, noticing those subtle signals. You can eat, enjoy and notice when you feel the 'I'm satisfied' feeling, and then thank the body and the mind, STOPPING when you know you do not need to eat any more.

When you are done and completely satisfied you can thank the body and the mind. What you may have been doing in the past is going into that

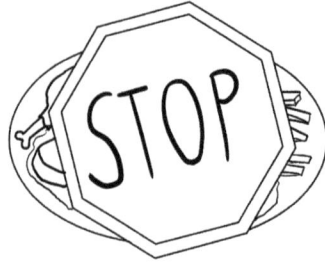

overly full mode when you continue to eat after you have received the 'I am satisfied' signal. You know the scenario where the stomach sends the message to the subconscious and the subconscious sends the message on to the conscious mind that you are full or satisfied and the conscious mind chooses to ignore that message, sending back the message that 'this is too nice to waste' and continues eating. What happens is, we often overeat until we feel like we are going to burst and then we wait 20 minutes and top it up again with sweets.

When you choose to ignore that initial signal and continue to keep eating until you are overfull, you become very uncomfortable. If you think about it, it is not a pleasant feeling at all and is really one that drains you of energy and is a feeling that you would rather not experience. You may find you actually want more food because of your old beliefs that you cannot throw away and waste food. The old belief can tell you that you have created space in the body, space that needs to be continually filled up again.

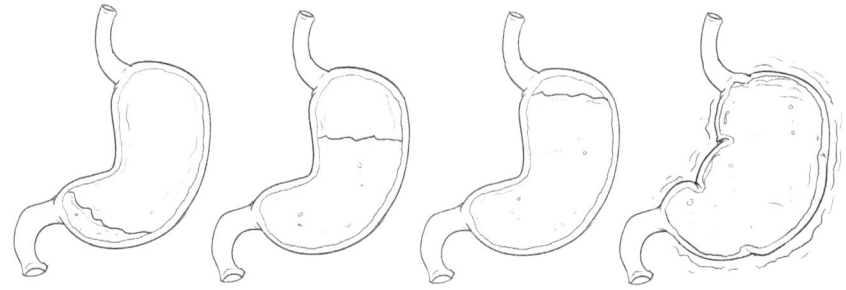

These are the old habits and behaviours we need to address and to stop. You have a choice whether to change old patterns or simply create new ones.

Discovering those reasons why you eat and uncovering unhealthy associations is an important part of this process.

Chapter 3
'Try' and 'Hope'

> If you find you are using food to 'fix' something, you may need to find other more suitable ways to deal with those emotions.

Emotional eating occurs when food becomes a source of comfort when you are feeling sad, lonely, bored, angry or even anxious. The craving for food can attach itself to many different emotions, often causing greater stress and discomfort. Food can even become an emotional trigger, causing you to feel more anxious or more stressed. Just like the Pavlov's dog theory of classical conditioning where Pavlov trained dogs to salivate at the mere ringing of a bell, we often form connections with food and emotions. For those of you who are not familiar with such an experiment, Ivan Petrovich Pavlov was a Russian Scientist back in the late 1800s, early 1900s, who was known for his impact in the field of physiology of mammals. He discovered unusual responses to drooling dogs through experiments that had identified true reactions that came from different stimuli which had nothing to do with food. We do not support testing on animals; however, we understand that back in those days discoveries were often made through uncommon trials (Fred, 2001). It is certainly not an era we would have liked to experience, as animals are just as sacred as the human species. We do apologise for referring to this information, however, we felt it necessary to share research based material when it applies to something so significant to programming the mind.

So the next time you find yourself reaching for food for emotional comfort, it may be fitting to ask yourself some of the following questions and note them in the NIB:

1. What was my trigger that sent me to the kitchen?
2. Am I truly physically hungry?
3. How do I feel physically or emotionally at this moment?
4. What is the emotional benefit of eating?
5. If I am not really hungry for food, what is it I really need?

You need to validate your feelings, make room for them, and make a choice to do something different other than eat. Remember, we do not need to fill our stomachs to gain control.

You may discover that you need something else other than food. If you feel sad, can you call a friend for emotional support? If you feel stressed, you could take a nice warm shower or bath, listen to some music or a relaxation meditation. The key is to acknowledge and validate the way you feel, make room for that feeling, and make a decision to do different and not to feed the mouth with food.

You can listen to soothing voices and music that best suits your needs. This helps the mind totally chill out and become free from the hustle and bustle of busy life. You are welcome to download a complimentary mindful meditation – simply go to our website www.CasTherapy.com, enter your name and email address and download the mp3 with our compliments.

If you feel anxious you could exercise or take a long walk to clear the mind. Food is not a reward for the body, food is merely sustenance for the body to give you the energy you need for the day. You can retrain the mind to believe a reward is treating yourself to a movie or doing something nice for yourself, like indulging in a massage, going for a walk or taking some time just for you to do something that is special and something you enjoy doing. Nurturing is all part of the process of self-respect which sends those messages to the brain that you are 'worth it' and deserve the best.

Emotions are a very collective eating trigger. If you find yourself continually turning to food instead of digging a little deeper for the underlying cause, you are not taking steps to resolve the core issue. Keeping a food journal may help you discover any emotional triggers that cause you to engage in unhealthy habits. Writing down what you eat can also help you see and make connections you may not have been aware of previously.

Let us examine some common reasons why you may eat when you are not truly hungry.

- You eat because other people are eating.
- You eat because food is present.
- You eat to celebrate a happy occasion like a birthday, graduation or anniversary.
- You eat because you are tired or cranky.
- You eat because the clock says it is time to eat.
- You eat because the food is cheap or even free.
- You eat because people are pushing you to eat.
- You eat because you feel the need to always clean your plate.

We live in a society that is centred around food. We celebrate with food, we commiserate with food and we eat when we are happy, sad, glad and mad. We often build our day around food, using food as a pacifier at times because it is easier than facing the raw emotions.

> When you discover and can learn to practise mindful eating, you can become one with the body and you can learn to appreciate and respect food, rather than always looking at food as the enemy or the crutch.

Practising mindful eating

According to the Harvard Health Letter (2011), mindful eating is based on the Buddhist concept of mindfulness, or being fully aware of what is happening within and around you at the moment (Mindful eating, 2011). Mindfulness promotes healthy eating and can also help relieve stress and even alleviate problems like high blood pressure and gastrointestinal issues (Weil, 2007).

What does 'mindfulness' really mean when it comes to eating healthy? Mindfulness when applied to eating is all about noticing the colours, the smells, the flavours and even the textures of foods. It is about eliminating distractions and really concentrating on the food at hand.

A study led by psychologist Jean Kristeller at Indiana State University and Duke University found that binge eaters who practised mindfulness-based therapy actually enjoyed their food more and found they had less of a sense of struggle when it came to controlling their eating (Baer, 2006). The study suggests that mindfulness helps one better recognise the difference between emotional and physical hunger and satiety because it helps discover that moment of choice between the urge to eat and eating.

The mouth, talks to the mind letting the brain know that food is coming. The mind goes into the thinking thought processes, listening, validating letting the mouth know that you are taking your time to decide what to eat and when to eat, and how much to eat, as you are in control of your choices.

The best way to practise mindful eating is to start by approaching to eat in a slower, more gradual way. You can even set a kitchen timer to 20 minutes, taking at least that long to eat and enjoy your meal.

You may choose to begin by eating silently for 5–10 minutes, taking time to contemplate what it took to produce the food you are eating. Imagine the path that your food took from the ground to the table and thank your food for the sustenance it provides you. When you allow the mind to really take the journey of the food to the table, you bring a whole new meaning to your relationship with food.

Notice how you are now eating to refuel the body. Eating is a separate activity and, as such, needs to be done by itself and not in conjunction with any other activity.

So... what we endorse is:

1. Drink a full glass of water 15 minutes prior to each meal. Sit down at the table for each of your meals (not at your desk, in the car or while you are on the run).

2. Knife and fork down between each mouthful, bringing awareness to the present.

3. Chew your food slowly; your teeth are in your mouth for a reason.

4. Notice the flavours, allow the tastebuds to do their work.

5. Stop halfway through your meal and ask 'Am I satisfied?' If you are, **STOP** and push your plate away.

6. Thank the body and the mind.

7. Notice the taste within the mouth and savour the flavour.

> Mindfulness is about eating slowly and respectfully, taking small bites and enjoying your food and chewing it thoroughly.

Many times eating too fast and eating while you are distracted or in a rush causes you to eat more than you really intend to and require, and being mindful can help you overcome that trait.

The Indian phrase known as 'rasa' literally means taste. To enhance your appreciation of 'rasa' means to cultivate your ability to really enjoy the taste, the flavour and the individual characteristics of food. When you eat in this manner, you digest your food more efficiently and you absorb the nutrients more effectively which means you feel satisfied much sooner.

This is another approach to mindful eating. You appreciate your food much more and it can help you make healthier choices. As you tune in to the 'rasa' of your food, you will soon discover the cravings that might have caused you to sabotage your healthy eating quickly disappearing, leading you to desire fresh, wholesome foods over unhealthy foods.

Brian Wansink, PhD, (2010) the director of Cornell Universities Food and Brand Lab, states that mindful eating is the key to healthy eating. He goes on to say that the average person makes over 250 decisions each day when it comes to food, and he found that many of us have no idea as to what influences our choices (Wansink, 2010).

Wansink (2010) completed an interesting experiment where he fixed a bottomless soup bowl which kept the bowl half full, no matter how much people ate. Participants who were served food in the bottomless bowls ate at least 15 ounces more than those who ate out of normal bowls.

Most likely you would have heard the saying 'my eyes are bigger than my stomach', which makes sense. We often think we are hungry, ravished in fact, when really we are only a little bit peckish. You will read more about 'perception' later as we continue to travel through the process of change. We also have the 'nose', the smell sense which activates the 'must have' signal, the one that you cannot say no to. The aromas are so strong and overpowering that they seem to direct you to a decision that creates the behaviour that you simply cannot resist. Remember, this is only one sense that has been activated and you have the inner power to validate and move on.

Cas gives an example about her experience with Vegemite toast and goes on to show you her conversation within her mind. 'Mmm, I love the smell of fresh hot toast steaming from the toaster; there is something about cooked bread. I love butter and Vegemite, how it soaks up into the toast, tasting tangy. What am I thinking, I don't even eat toast.'

Cas' mind goes into the imagination side where she dreams of toast being smothered with Vegemite ready to eat. Now, Cas believed that this was truly a memory for her, as she has not eaten toast and Vegemite for many years, yet the sensation was so strong. It was like it was only yesterday and the craving was very powerful.

You see, the mind will check in with you to see what your truth is now – 'Do I eat that sort of food or is it only a memory?' You need to slow down the thought process and check in with self to actually reflect on what is truly occurring. Do not be fooled by memories; just allow the mind to come into your current choices and what matters most. Your mind may create those memories and flag the emotions that are attached to those memories as if they were valid and real today. If those emotions are not useful or helpful, then make the decision to leave those emotions with their memories, leaving them in the past.

What all this is telling us is that visual cues such as your surroundings and even your eating companions can help you eat in a more mindful manner. When you become more mindful and start eating more slowly and expressing more gratitude and more appreciation for your food, you begin to pay more attention to those feelings of fullness. You begin to focus more on those subtle cues that trigger in the mind and the stomach the feeling that you are satiated. When you listen to your senses, the aromas and visuals, a part of your mind will take you to your current choices of how and what to eat.

Being one with the body

Really understanding the needs of your body and mind can take some exploration. A reality check of basic human needs can help you identify your true needs, not just your wants.

> Reality therapy teaches that we need NOT be victims of our past, our present and our external forces that surround us, unless we choose to be (Glasser, 1998).

Being one with the body means to be connected with the body. According to Dr William Glasser, being disconnected is the source of almost all human problems (Glasser, 1998). Glasser talks about the 'Seven Caring Habits' in Choice Theory: supporting, encouraging, listening, accepting, trusting, respecting and negotiating the differences. These axioms describe the perfect scenario and relationship between the mind and the body. When you learn to respect the body and become one with the body, you can make better choices, choices that support a healthy, vibrant body.

It is important to remember why you eat to begin with. You eat to refuel the body and you eat so you can do all the things you choose to do like walking, working, playing and having fun.

Glasser articulates that the mind and the body default back to fulfilling your five basic human needs:

1. Survival, shelter, sex.

2. Love and belonging.

3. Power, self and self-control.

4. Freedom, free to choose.

5. Fun, pleasure and enjoyment.

All of your behaviours are driven to meet these needs. Every time you do something there is a force that drives that behaviour towards an unmet need, thus the focus is on what is actually missing in your life and/or are your needs being met (Glasser, 1998). If they are not being met then steps need to be taken to identify your needs so you can make the choices to do different, meeting the needs that best suit your values and your lifestyle.

Chapter 3
'Try' and 'Hope'

ACTIVITY 7: MEETING FIVE NEEDS
How do you meet the 5 Basic Needs?

1. _____

2. _____

3. _____

4. _____

5. _____

Take your time.

Choice Theory also suggests that the only person whose behaviour you can control is your own (Glasser, 1998). Choice Theory infers that what happened to you in the past has everything to do with who you are today, however you can only satisfy your basic needs in the here and now. What we believe this means is that yesterday is done and gone. The choices you made in the past as it pertains to food may have created the body you live in today, you can change the body you create for tomorrow by making different and better choices from this moment forward. You have the power to make those choices.

When you choose to chew slowly and spend the time to actually taste the food, you put less pressure on the stomach and on the body. If you swallow the food prior to chewing, it can actually traumatise the body by causing the stomach to labour and work much harder. You ultimately have the power to create, to make and do different. That power belongs to you and only you can make that power connect and commit to all that you desire.

Understanding the job your stomach undertakes can only influence your decisions to do different. Our body relies on the input of healthy food and clean water for it to work efficiently. It is simply not the role of the stomach to just process your food. Your stomach's role is to digest and extract the nutrients and redirect them to specific places within the body. The stomach has a clever way of ensuring that your body is fed what it needs to function effectively. This is the reason why we need to nourish and supply our bodies with healthy, nutritious foods (quality fuel). When you develop the habit of placing the knife and fork down in between each mouthful and you spend the time being mindful of your food by tasting and enjoying the textures, you enjoy the process of eating much more. If you are eating in front of the television or during any other activity, that needs to change, as you have decided to be healthy and live a healthy lifestyle. Often we do not know how much we eat when we are busy watching television and staring at the pictures. Having awareness keeps the focus on being and living healthy every day and making a conscious decision to live in the present – enjoying those present decisions that make your life FUN.

This is also a good time to consider a hobby or other kind of activity, especially if you had been eating out of boredom before. Remember, as soon as you notice those signals within the body, stop and take notice. Stop when you are comfortable, stop when you are satisfied and thank the body and the mind, as they do all the hard work. You know your body and mind better than anyone else, so take the time to listen and connect to those messages.

If you have found yourself at the cupboard, swinging on the handles, saying things to yourself like: 'There is nothing to eat in here', 'I am not really hungry', 'Ah, that will do', as you grab a bag of something to munch on, the message is loud and clear. You need to find something else to do. It is time to do different and it is time to listen to what those parts of you are telling you. Stop! What is it your mind is really telling you? What is the underlying message? You clearly are not hungry and you are looking for food to fill some other type of void. Remember, you have the power to choose, utilise the '**Choice Power**' pathway and make the decisions that are useful and helpful to live in an overall healthy manner.

> When you make the decision to be true to you and the decision to be the person you choose to be, it is much easier to maintain a healthy lifestyle.

It is important to trust the process – to have faith in yourself – to remove the fear. Know your values and beliefs because they are your foundations.

Action: Remove the words 'try' and 'hope' from your vocabulary. If you look back on your life, being honest with yourself, anytime you tried to do something, YOU FAILED. If you look back at your life, anytime you have said to yourself 'I'm going to do it' and there was no question about it, you did it, and you possibly did it very well. 'Hope' and 'try' are twins and 'try' means automatic failure. If you eliminate the words 'hope' and 'try' from your vocabulary from this moment on, you are going to notice a difference immediately.

So be clear with yourself and ask yourself, 'Is this taking me in the direction I want to go – Yes or No? And if 'No,' 'Am I ready, willing and able to accept those consequences?' We suggest using crisp, clear, clean language like 'I am', 'I will' or 'I chose' in order to give yourself clear direction.

Hey Hey It's Me!

ACTIVITY 8: THOUGHT STOPPING BAND
Reasons why I may *subconsciously* *choose* to hold on to excess weight:

To make this a habit, we suggest placing a rubber band or something similar around your wrist (not too tight) and every time you hear yourself say one of those words, flick the band. This is called a 'thought stopping technique' and can be useful to change unwanted thoughts. Many therapists utilise thought stopping techniques which stem from Cognitive Behavioural Therapy (CBT). CBT is a powerful tool to change the conscious thoughts and patterns of behaviour and works really well with reality theory. According to Edelman our 'cognitions are made up of thoughts and beliefs' (Edelman, 2006, p. 6), however, they are very different and need to be addressed differently. When you are utilising the thought stopping technique you allow the mind to 'stop, think and change', reset the thinking pattern and away you go. Within a short amount of time you will have removed those words completely and you will be noticing the changes in your life.

Sadly, the word 'try' will become like a terrible swear word to you. As soon as someone mentions the word you will notice it and observe that they are not committed to you or to the task at hand.

Stay tuned, we will be adding more words to the flick band as we progress. You do not have to utilise the band technique; it is only a tool that some like to use, hence the reason we have included it. We often use a 'click' of the fingers for each time you want a thought change. It is easy and works just as well and you can do it without anyone noticing. Choose what works for you and what you find useful and helpful.

Chapter 4

Diet Versus a Healthy Lifestyle

What do you say to yourself when you hear the word 'diet'?

As we discussed in the first chapter, the word 'diet' has a very negative connotation. What do you think of when you say or hear the word diet? The word 'diet' often has no energy and no enthusiasm, and can infer deprivation. It sends the message that you cannot have something or that you need to deprive yourself of something. It sends the message that it is too hard or it takes too much effort. The word 'diet' may even cause you to want to slump over in your chair lacking in energy.

> The word 'diet' is NOT a cause for celebration. The term healthy lifestyle has energy and enthusiasm.

ACTIVITY 9: DIET VS HEALTHY LIFESTYLE

We would like you to stop for a moment, take a piece of paper and place a line down the centre of the paper. At the top of the left hand column write the word 'diet'. Now spend a couple of minutes writing down under the word everything you can think of and everything you feel about going on a diet.

Welcome back...

What did you think and feel about going on a diet? Many people instantly respond with 'No more yummy foods' or 'All I can eat is salads, steamed veggies and lettuce leaves'. You may have thought of someone being forced to eat foods that they did not really like or want.

Now... think of a colour you would associate with the word 'diet'. What would that colour be? It is likely you would think of a shade of black or grey. Some people may have their least favourite colour spring to mind or the colour red, stating it represents that they have to stop. So when you think of the word 'diet', it is often not very positive and can actually be quite draining. The word just does not feel energising or exciting.

When you think of going on a 'diet' it might bring to mind restrictive meal plans or even bestselling books by overly slim and often Photoshopped celebrities. One might also think of 'guilt producing health nuts' who attempt to make you feel bad about yourself.

For those who may have been diagnosed with a weight related illness, like Type 2 Diabetes or metabolic syndrome, the word 'diet' might bring to mind a healthcare professional harassing you, which may not be the most inspiring image. The word 'diet' just seems like a lot of hard work for someone who is already very busy. The thought of a diet can be downright draining. There is already way too much talk about diets. As a matter of fact, it may seem like everyone you know is on a diet or has been on a diet at some time or another.

'Losing weight' and 'diet' language is what keeps the 'Weight Loss' industry in business. This language simply keeps recycling big people and yoyo dieters, up and down, to lose and find the weight again. The industry is often programming (unknowingly) people to fail by feeding the subconscious mind language that is confusing, giving unclear direction. Diets simply do not work long term. As we have said, this book is not about a diet. It is about giving you a system and guidelines to adopt a physical and mental healthy lifestyle. It is about being, living, eating,

Chapter 4
Diet Versus a Healthy Lifestyle

feeling and thinking healthy long term and addressing or identifying issues that are possibly the cause of you being held back in the past.

> ## WHAT DO YOU THINK OF WHEN YOU SAY OR HEAR THE WORDS 'HEALTHY LIFESTYLE'?
>
> Again, stop for a few minutes. Pick up that piece of paper on which you have already written what you think and feel about being on a diet. Write the words 'healthy lifestyle' as a heading in the right hand column. Again, place the book down and spend a few minutes writing down everything you think and feel about living a healthy lifestyle.

Again welcome back...

Now, what did you think when you thought about living a healthy lifestyle? Often people move in their seats, they sit up straighter, smile and a new part of them that is way more interested in this process becomes obvious. The first answers are often similar to statements like: 'I am going to be healthier', 'I am going to have more energy', 'I will be happier', and 'I will be able to live longer'.

The phrase 'healthy lifestyle' has much more energy and enthusiasm. It makes you want to sit up straight and pay attention. It feels lighter and brighter. You may have equated the phrase 'healthy lifestyle' to a bright and sunny day, out having fun, enjoying the warmth and fresh air, being with the people you love and care about. You might think of people who have a smile on their face or people exercising or playing a sport, or maybe just running around the park.

How did you articulate a healthy lifestyle? If you had to associate a colour with a 'healthy lifestyle', what colour would that be? You may have thought of yellow or green, or perhaps some other light and bright colour, or you may have thought of your favourite colour. You might even think of a colourful meadow with beautiful flowers.

> The term healthy lifestyle can bring to mind bright and colourful surroundings filled with creative images that the imagination projects.

One very obvious difference we have noticed in doing this exercise over the years with many of our clients is that it is highly likely that you may not have even thought about or mentioned food at all when thinking of living a healthy lifestyle, as compared to the thinking on the other side of the paper, which is often focused around food and deprivation.

Therefore, the term 'healthy lifestyle' is a more positive term both mentally and physically. So from this point on repeat to yourself many times per day, loudly and passionately, 'I am NOW living a healthy lifestyle and I always WILL!' You can yell this from the rooftops if you choose, or you can imagine yourself yelling it from the rooftops silently within your subconscious mind. Just be sure to repeat it often, with conviction.

When you choose to live a healthy lifestyle, you feel better about yourself. You are making a conscious choice to choose better health. You are taking a new road. Most people, if given the choice, would choose a healthy lifestyle over an unhealthy one.

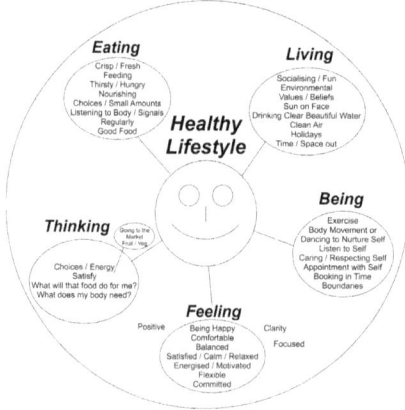

Action: Words to add to the 'not to be used language' are: 'Diet' and 'Lose Weight' or any other term that refers to 'losing' or 'lost'. Flick that band, every time you hear yourself use those words. And if someone comes up to you, saying, 'Hey you look great and healthy, have you lost weight?' simply reply with, 'Thanks, I have thrown it away and I feel

Chapter 4
Diet Versus a Healthy Lifestyle

fantastic.' You are now living, thinking, being, eating and feeling healthy. Refer to the Healthy Lifestyle circle diagram. (There is a larger version of the diagram on page 90.)

Food as fuel – the sports car analogy

When you begin to look at food as fuel, it changes your thinking. We like to use the analogy of the red sports car once again.

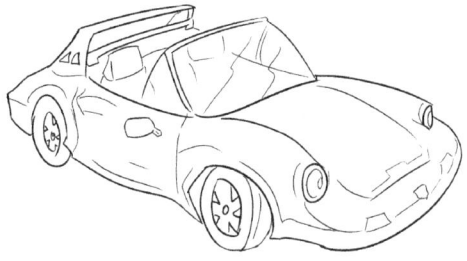

When you think of the body like a fine sports car it changes the way you think and the way you feel.

If you drove an expensive sports car, you would treat it with the utmost respect. You would not put the wrong fuel into it. You would only fill it with the finest fuel. You would take the time to clean it, polish it and keep it in tip-

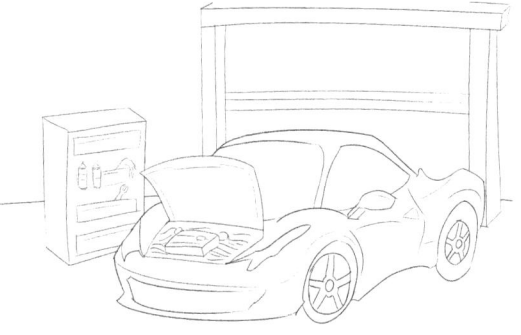

top condition. You would not abuse the car or drive a filthy car around. You would be very proud to drive this sports car, so you would do what it takes to maintain the car with the best possible care.

Just as the proper fuel keeps a car running smoothly, healthy nutritious food keeps the body running smoothly. The body is a work of art, your work of art. When you think of food as fuel, it changes the way you think and the way you eat. It helps you make better choices because you feel good about those choices. Everything you eat fuels the body. If you eat poorly, then the body runs poorly. If you eat in a healthy manner, the body thrives.

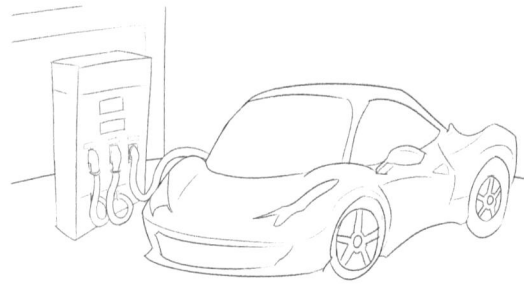

It is also highly unlikely that you would drive your sports car to a petrol station, fill it to full and then continue pumping, because that would be a waste, dangerous and rather messy. So do the same with your body. It is your vehicle to carry you through life, so fill it to a satisfactory level and stop. If you think about it, it would be waste one way or another, waste as in leftovers to put back in the cupboard, the fridge or the rubbish bin. Or waste, as over-consumed food that has got to go somewhere and ends up on your waist or your butt. So you see, either way it is waste. And you are not the rubbish bin.

This process and system is about learning new behaviours. Now remember that the new habits and behaviours we are creating are EASY creations and learnings that need to be repeated over and over again. Repetition, like anything else in our lives, creates confidence and security. When you repeat something often enough it becomes a new program within the mind, a new habit that appears to be automatic and done without effort. For example, when you drive a European car and the indicator is on the opposite side to what you are used to, you go around a few corners turning on the wipers instead of the indicator. However, it does not take long for you to learn you are not achieving the desired outcome and you adapt quickly to utilising the lever on the opposite side of the steering wheel. Thus, the experience teaches us quickly that to obtain the desired results we need to adjust our behaviours.

When you start to live a healthier lifestyle you start to eliminate old behaviours. For example, do you eat in front of the television? If so,

Chapter 4
Diet Versus a Healthy Lifestyle

one of the first modifications to make is to eliminate eating in front of the television. Eating is actually a separate behaviour – we eat to refuel the body and television is a form of entertainment. When you eat in front of the television or the computer, you are not even conscious of what or how much you are putting into your mouth because the activity is secondary. Your body deserves time and attention as it is being refuelled, so that you become aware of when it is satisfied and when it is time to stop. You are not too busy for you. There are 24 hours in a day and you deserve some of that time to look after and nurture yourself. Again, think of your body as your vehicle; you would not take your car to a petrol station, fill it to full, then drive to the next station and top it up, followed by the next station and the next and the next. However, that is what we often do when we eat mindlessly.

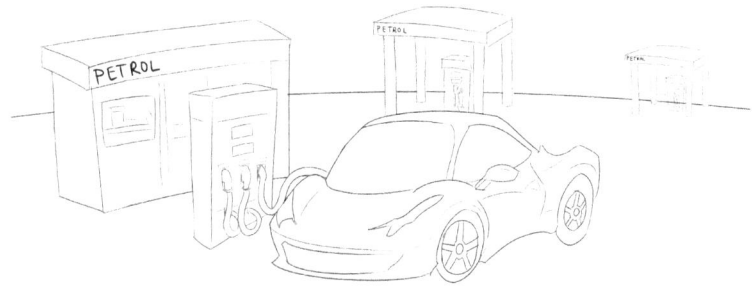

We must be very clear when we are communicating with the mind. Any kind of eating, including snacks, we suggest be eaten at the dining room or the kitchen table. Every time you eat in the car or on the run, again, you are telling the mind you are too busy to stop and nourish the body, and you are not worth it, so the mind believes that you think that you are not important.

When you know and decide to live a healthy lifestyle you are always aware of yourself and the direction in which you choose to go. Therefore, if for some reason you happen to stray, it is easy to get yourself back on track, because you simply know the long-term direction in which you choose to live. When you have a clear path to follow, with no 'hopes' and 'tries' you always know where you are going. When you choose the road to better health, you have a firm plan to follow and a good solid foundation. You treat yourself and the body with respect, and the body rewards you.

Eating to live versus living to eat

When you eat to live rather than live to eat, it changes your perspective. When you view food as fuel, junk food becomes insignificant and less important. When you view the body as your temple, you want to feed it nourishing, healthy foods because they give you more energy and you feel better. Life is meant to be enjoyed and the central focus of life is likely better for you if it does not revolve solely around food. There is much more to life than food. Do not worry, we are not intending to take away the enjoyment of the food you do eat; in fact, with mindful eating, it is intended that this new found awareness will actually allow you to become very aware of what you eat and, therefore, it is likely that this awareness will increase your enjoyment level.

When you shift your thinking from food as 'comfort' to food as sustenance, you begin to view food differently. You make better, healthier choices. You begin to live your life in a healthier manner. You do not go to a party to enjoy the 'food', you go to enjoy the people and the surroundings. It is important not to test yourself when you go to a party. Make a conscious decision not to stand by the food table – that way if you are going to eat it is a conscious decision and not a mindless pick up and eat during a social conversation. If you stray a little and make a choice to indulge every once in a while, then that is okay too, as long as you are aware of the choices and the consequences. With this awareness you are likely to return quickly and continue on a healthy pathway.

> When you view the body as your vehicle, it changes the way you think and feel at a very deep level of the mind.

Chapter 4
Diet Versus a Healthy Lifestyle

One of the most important factors in all of this is WATER. Up to 60% of the human adult body is water and water cleanses the system, hydrates the organs and rejuvenates the skin. Water is the potion of life and it helps you feel energised and alive. When you drink water, you clear the body of impurities. As you drink water imagine that it is travelling through the body cleansing the cells and collecting the fat from the cells and then imagine that water carrying all of that mass, those toxins and poisons, and disposing of it, releasing it and throwing it away out of your system. Water is the key to a healthy lifestyle because without it you cannot thrive and you certainly cannot survive.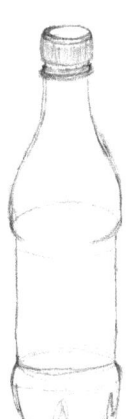

Those who live to eat look at food as much more than just fuel. They might look at food as an emotional release or look at food as comfort. Someone who lives to eat gives food a greater meaning than merely a nutritional value. When food begins to take on a much greater meaning than sustenance, you start running into conflicting desires and commitments from different parts within the mind that are seeking some other type of security, satisfaction or need that the part is looking to fill. Food then begins to drive your emotions and your desires which can be misplaced, disruptive and destructive.

When you eat to live, as our system here is guiding you through the steps to do now, you make a healthy and positive choice to live a better life. Food becomes fuel, nothing more and nothing less. You begin to take pride in the healthy food you choose to ingest.

> When you give the body what it needs through proper nutrition, you feel better about yourself.

When you mindfully eat healthy, you become more self-aware of what it is you put into and do to the body. It helps to think of the body as your vehicle. If you allow the vehicle to run out of fuel, the vehicle will not run. If you feed and maintain the vehicle with the correct amounts, it runs

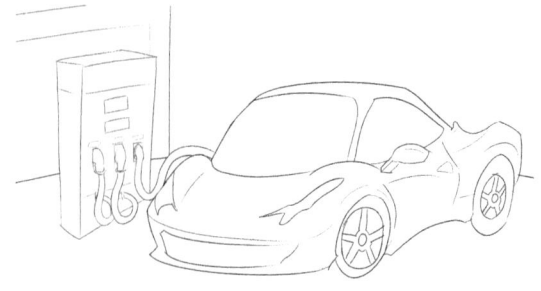

smoothly and efficiently. If it is maintained and fuelled correctly it is likely it will grow to be a valuable vintage model that continues to work and function perfectly. Therefore, we hope the analogy of your body being your vehicle to carry you through your life will assist you in also growing to be a valuable vintage model, one that continues to function effectively.

When you eat to live you take pride in feeding the body what it needs to thrive and you will find many things on many different levels begin to improve. Food is no longer an addiction, it's simply a joy. You begin to enjoy simple healthy foods. You eat real, whole foods in a healthier manner and realise that when you eat in this way, you literally feel better and more alive. You are what you eat, in every sense of the word.

We have previously talked about the struggle that can occur between mind and body and the relationship with food that we have. A wonderful strategy within this chapter can switch the 'struggle' off permanently, enhancing your way of thinking and feeling within the relationship that you are now developing with food.

> When you eat unhealthy, overly processed foods, the body is bogged down. When you eat real whole foods and foods that are healthy and nutrient dense, the body feels better and has more energy.

Food cannot only help you live a better life, it may also help you live a longer life. Thanks to the antioxidants that natural food provides, food can actually have some incredible health benefits. The simple processes of eating and breathing, which are common everyday processes, produce what are called free radicals, which are dangerous substances in the body, substances that can actually eat away at healthy cells (Shurkin, 2004). When you feed the body natural, whole, nutrient dense foods that contain antioxidants, it can counteract this damage.

In 2004, Shurkin referred to particular foods, such as green foods like broccoli, kale and Swiss chard, which help to fend off both macular degeneration and cataracts, while garlic can actually help you lower cholesterol.

Foods like spinach contain lutein, a substance that blocks blue light. This can damage the macula or the part of the eye that enables you to see fine details (Shurkin, 2004).

Shurkin (2004) also mentions teas like black and green tea which contain bioflavonoids called catechins. Green tea contains a powerful antioxidant that has been shown to be helpful in preventing degenerative brain disease.

Brussels sprouts, those tiny little adorable cabbages, also share the same wonderful healing properties that other cruciferous vegetables have and they are high in fibre and antioxidants and rich in vitamin C (Shurkin, 2004).

Celery is both an appetite suppressant and a natural source of electrolytes and can act as a natural tranquilliser for insomniacs. Tolman (NaturalNews, 2012), the Whole Food Medicine Cowboy who is a catalyst for natural and ancient remedies, reports that celery is also good for the bones. Cranberries have long been known for their medicinal qualities and have been used for many years to help fight urinary tract infections.

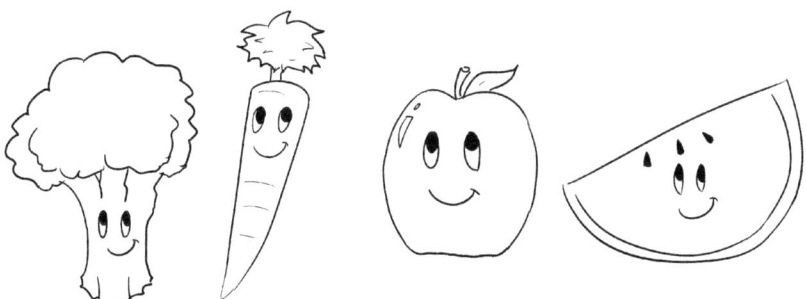

Cucumbers are high in silica, a substance that helps strengthen the body's connective tissues. Phytonutrients are natural compounds found in plants and scientists have proven that these compounds help protect plants and help them survive, and they can also do the same for humans. Also known as phytochemicals, they contain amazing restorative properties, some of which we are still discovering. The colours in fruits and vegetables help plants attract pollinators and these same colours can help humans heal, prevent illness and even slow the aging process!

> Fruit and vegetables are our best friends. They are with us every single day, week, month and year to help support us and guide us to live a richer, meaningful life. Like a best friend, they listen, they feed and validate in ways that we may never fully understand.

Tolman looked into all kinds of ancient archives before stumbling across the signature science of the nature of food, being the law of similarity. If the food looks like an organ in the body, it targets that specific organ. The food itself is good for the whole body by increasing the capacity and function of that particular organ, for instance walnuts look like the brain, with left and right hemispheres, the convoluted wrinkles on the nut just like the neocortex (NaturalNews, 2012).

These are just a few simple examples of the power of natural food and there are many more. Natural food gives you that mental edge and it not only helps you maintain your ideal weight, it also can help you live a better life.

In the end, life is more than any given therapy – it is about lifestyle and taking the appropriate steps to become healthy, and eating healthy nutritious food is certainly the key to a healthy lifestyle.

Chapter 4
Diet Versus a Healthy Lifestyle

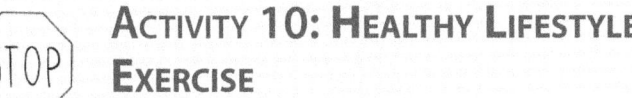

ACTIVITY 10: HEALTHY LIFESTYLE EXERCISE

Imagine a light switch, or a lever or something that you can turn on in the subconscious mind. Now gently close your eyes and access the imagination and say the following with passion and conviction:

'I am **NOW** living a healthy lifestyle and I always **WILL**' and as you say the word 'will' in your subconscious mind, imagine that you are easily flicking on that switch.

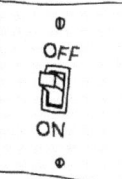

Say those words over and over again 15 or 20 times per day – say them and repeat them over and over. By doing this you are reprogramming the subconscious mind. This becomes your new mantra, your new way of life.

'I am **NOW** living a healthy lifestyle and I always **WILL**.' Remember, you have the power to switch the struggle off and switch on the light that connects you to living a healthy lifestyle. ***'Whatever the mind creates, the mind can heal and change.'***

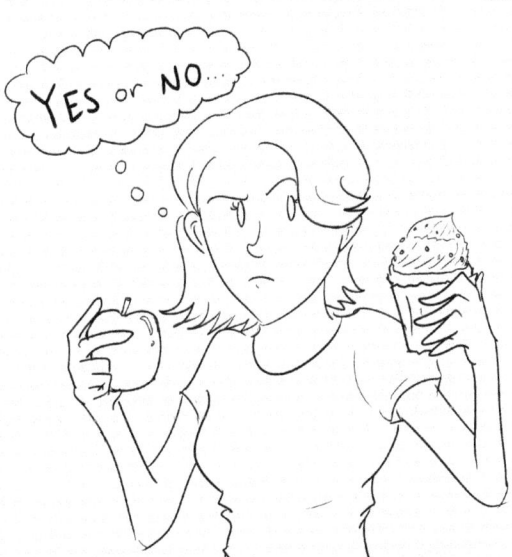

Living a healthy life, you decide, you are your own authority of the mind, and you make your choices about your life.

89

The Circle to Health

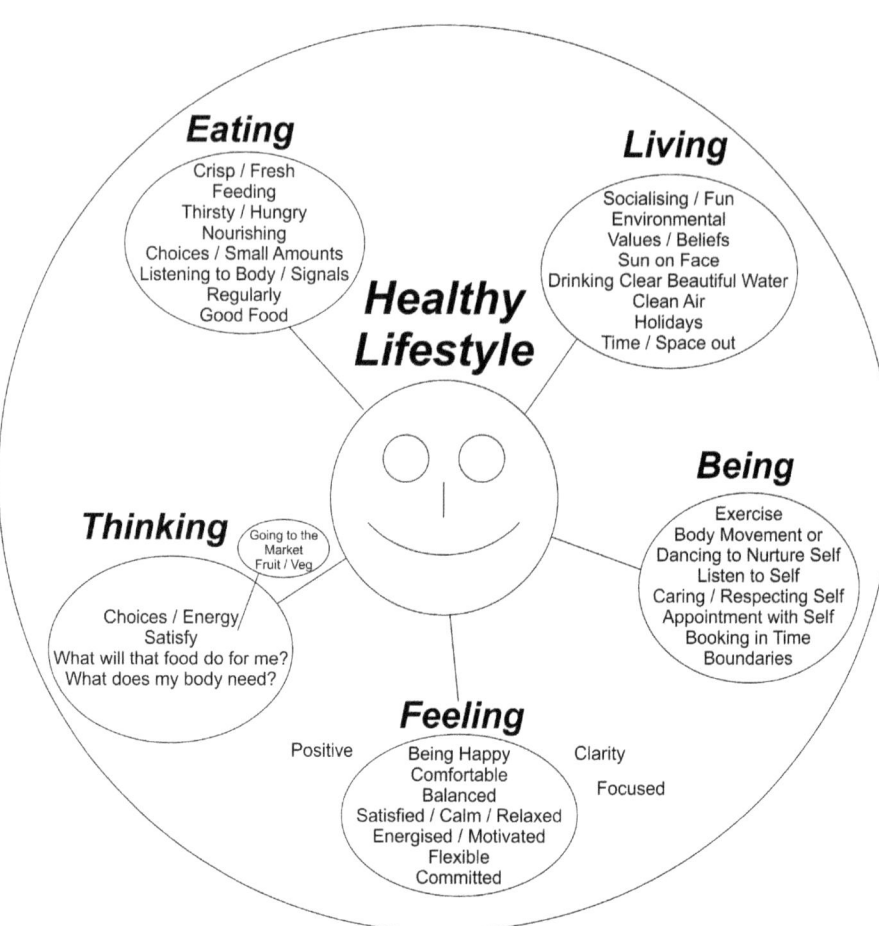

Chapter 5

Eating and Your Emotions

The emotional connection with food

In order to understand how to control your emotions you must first understand what an emotion is and where it is formed. Humans revel in emotion and without emotions life would be very dull. When it comes down to it, emotions are necessary for a rich and fulfilling life. We live and breathe by our emotions and emotions make life worth living.

It is important to realise that YOU are NOT your emotions. Your emotions stem from your ego and if you can learn to separate yourself from your emotions and understand the positive intent behind them, you can change how you view the emotion. This concept is also known as '**reframing**'. Reframing comes under CBT which makes up part of the thoughts change process. This type of reframing allows a person to look through new lenses in a more constructive way that is useful and helpful (Edelman, 2006).

Let's have a look at how thoughts and feelings affect people on a conscious and subconscious level.

Humans are emotional beings with thoughts and feelings. What sets them apart from other creations is that they were given the gift of 'free will'. This 'free will' is used and exercised daily in making minor and major decisions in life. What influences the will is a dynamic process that involves thoughts and feelings and the conscious and subconscious mind. The 'free will' incorporates a pathway that allows the mind to make choices in our everyday life. This simply means that a human being has the choice to stay in bed or not to stay in bed, to say hello or not speak at all. So 'free will' allows that '**choice power**' part of that person to choose what they eat, when they eat and how much they eat. Keep in mind that a person's choice can depend on their feelings and emotions.

Understanding the human mind is a complex process that needs knowledge of the structure and the mental faculties involved in its function. The structure of the human brain can be briefly described as the master clock of the human body. It is the only structure that is directly linked with the functioning of all the other organs in the body. This is why people who lose their brain function are considered clinically dead and eventually lose all physical, mental and emotional sensations.

There are specific faculties of the brain that are associated with a person's cognitive functions. The frontal lobe controls thinking and judgment and the temporal lobe involves memory, dreams and emotions.

Theorist, Gordon Emmerson PhD, focuses on the theory of 'Ego State Therapy'. This theoretical framework is 'based on the premise that personality is composed of separate parts, rather than being a homogenous whole' (Emmerson, 2009, p. 1). These individual parts are developed as ego states.

As children develop, they learn to distinguish between what is beneficial and what is not helpful. Through responses and reactions to experiences these ego states develop and associate various emotions to particular situations which form the behaviours of the executive ego state. A good example would be a child who excels in class, who is constantly encouraged and motivated by his/her parents. This child will form happy thoughts and emotions which later may become their motivational ego state. On the other hand, a child who is constantly ridiculed and embarrassed for their actions may develop a protective ego state, which could surface at any time the child feels they need to be protected. The behaviour of the protective ego state could be defensive or destructive resulting in patterns of behaviour that do not suit the situation.

Hypnotherapy and ego state therapy allow a person to focus on the different ego states determining which are helpful and which are not. Through focusing and dissociation an individual can identify the ego states that need to change to bring about effective behavioural patterns.

According to Gordon Emmerson, PhD, (2009) ego states are actual parts of real feelings and emotions that play an important role on how the mind performs. Emmerson says that the ego states of a person remain inactive inside the mind until an event or situation activates it to come forward into the conscious executive state. The ego states of a person are numerous and involve various feelings and emotions. There are certain instances when they become intertwined or they may switch roles, depending on the circumstances involved. So in an actual setup, if a person experiences happy experiences, the happy ego states resurface and in the same manner. If a person experiences painful experiences, the sad ego states become evident. Depending upon the ego state present, or as the ego state therapist would call in an 'executive state', the emotion belonging to that state will influence the decision to eat healthy, to choose sweets, fatty foods or whatever that state feels desirable and more comfortable with.

In the same manner that helpful ego states are developed by a repetition of happy experiences, there can be disruptive ego states that, if not used properly, can cause a person to feel unhappy and therefore experience feelings of anger, fear, frustration etc. Interestingly, ego states have the ability to communicate with each other, creating an avenue to turn disruptive ego states into those that can be appropriately used by an individual.

In summary, the development of thoughts and feelings involves dynamic processes that are unique to each individual and are highly influenced by several factors such as childhood experiences, role models and events that occur throughout your lifetime.

You may not be able to change what is happening around you, however you can change how you 'react' or how you perceive each situation. Taking steps to understand the positive intent behind an emotion may help you better manage your emotions. You have the ability to respond and not react, it is simply a choice.

Many people have learnt to equate food with an emotional connection soon after birth because they may have experienced love and nurturing every time they were fed as a child. We often eat to socialise, nurture, express love and even eat to have fun. Generally speaking, in the Western world food is abundant and plentiful and many people use food to add pleasure and joy to their lives. While there is certainly nothing wrong with using food to celebrate happy occasions of life, emotional eating can become a problem if it is used to cope with or to avoid feelings and emotions. Food can then be programmed to be the crutch, the drug of choice to soothe all emotions.

Society has spread the idea that food is obtainable in first world countries at any opportunity, so why then do we experience the deprivation that drives us to despair and to either over or under eat?

John Gray, PhD, in *The Mars and Venus Diet and Exercise Solution*, talks about the importance of a balanced meal which places the body in a state of equilibrium where energy is maintained at a high level until the next food intake (Gray, 2003). This is the ultimate state of nutrition because you are eating to refuel the body and give the body a proper energy source.

This is the state of health we are striving for when we focus on being, living, eating, feeling and thinking healthy.

> When you eat real, natural, whole foods that nourish the body, you have endless energy and you feel more motivated to live a healthy life.

Chapter 5
Eating and Your Emotions

When you choose to eat nutritional foods that the body needs, you feel happier and more balanced. Gray comments that this kind of 'unconditional happiness means things make you happy and big problems don't knock you over' (Gray, 2003, p. 29). When you stop using foods as emotional comfort you are not dependent on food to fill in the gaps of your life. Eating proper foods improves your relationship with food and also balances brain chemistry, enabling you to see the whole picture, one that fits within your values and avoids focusing on the undesirable. Your whole mindset changes for the better! What this means is that 'No matter how bad things become, there are still many things to be grateful for' (Gray, 2003, p. 30).

Have you ever experienced wonderful feelings of peace and calmness, where those feelings came over your entire body, transporting waves of pleasure that you perhaps thought you could never experience again? You might have experienced it in water, swimming, floating or bathing. That same sensation can come just from feeling the freedom that you can incorporate into your life by making your own choices. That's exactly what can occur when you start to apply the elements of balance within your way of thinking and doing.

We like to equate that particular feeling with the experience of processing emotions and feeling the emotions instead of attempting to push them away, ignore them or cover them up with food.

Graham Park (2009), author of the book *7 Secrets the Weight Loss Industry Will Never Tell You*, refers to the fact that you are the driver of your choices and weight management can be easy and enjoyable rather than painful. Park believed that 'you have developed a habit of seeing food as the *problem* and not the solution (which it actually is)' (Park, 2009, p. 114). We have also identified that many people believe that food is their enemy, haunting them every day. You can live without smoking and drinking alcohol, you cannot live without food or water. So being told what to eat and what not to eat is unhelpful when you are on the weight management journey. Understanding the importance of food and what food can do for you is more helpful and most likely to inspire the journey of weight management. Simply utilising the philosophy that food is your solution makes sense when you actually reflect on the truth about healthy eating. Placing processed and synthetic products into our bodies can only create a false sense of balance. The whole idea about healthy eating is to go back to basics. Raw and natural foods can only do the body good. We believe that the process of weight management needs to be something you enjoy, rather than dread, that comes logically to you, because it feels natural and comfortable.

According to Park, nearly 6 million Australians engage the services of a weight management industry expert each year and, of those 6 million, 80% fail to follow through with a suggested program (2009).

Park also states that 95% of these people regained their weight within twelve months (Park, 2009). We do not want you to become a part of that statistic and by continuing to embark on this process together, we can overcome these old ways of behaviour, old patterns, old habits and associations together.

Practising feeling your emotions

Just how do you feel an emotion, you might ask. Riding emotional waves can be a transformative experience. It is non-productive to push emotions away because dealing with them as they arise allows you to move through them quickly. Emotions are simply clues that you can use to better understand your interpretation of an experience. You can work to identify those triggers that may cause you to overeat. When you establish a healthy emotional connection to food, you quickly realise that this too shall pass.

There are ways to bring the emotions back into balance and it is easier than you might think. You can have compassion for yourself and still feel the emotions. You can respond instead of reacting. When you discover how to feel the feelings and process and make room for those emotions instead of reacting to the emotions, you avoid labelling the emotions as good, bad, positive or negative.

Chapter 5
Eating and Your Emotions

We often judge our emotions, calling them good or bad, right or wrong, when we need to understand that emotions stem from feelings. People experience a feeling which can turn into an emotion, one that they might not be able to manage. For example, if a person feels sad, the feeling is 'sad'. That feeling may stay for a few moments or minutes and then simply fade away, or the feeling may become stronger, growing into an emotion and expressing a need to be heard in many ways. The 'sad' feeling becomes the emotional feeling of sadness, bouts of extreme sadness that might exhibit tears or anxiousness.

In *How to End Mindless Eating and Enjoy a Balanced Relationship with Food*, Susan Albers says many people turn to food when challenging or difficult feelings arise (Albers, 2012). Albers infers that emotional eating only stuffs down the emotions, not allowing the feelings to be processed. As a result the emotions consume you and can leave you feeling miserable (2012).

For example, if someone is doing something that annoys you, he/she does not make you angry. You choose to allow that behaviour to upset you. Someone else may find the exact same behaviour funny and that is simply their choice. Therefore, if you feel that emotion arising within you, it is a clue that you may wish to look closer at your experiences and explore why you react or respond in that particular way. If you do not like the response, what can you do different to alter that response? A great question to ask self is 'What is going on for me now?' Wait and listen to the answer. Your mind is clever and it will assist you if you ask.

In order to manage and process emotions, we have compiled a list of suggestions that may help with bringing about your self-awareness. Take your time to answer while you allow yourself to go through this process and write in your journal or NIB.

Activity 11: Learning and Exploring Emotions

- Identify your emotions and observe how you are feeling. Write down the emotions in your journal or NIB. (It is a good idea to combine an emotions journal with the food diary. This way you are able to follow any patterns that may be present. Record what you had for lunch and at dinner time, and record how you felt throughout the afternoon.) You do not have to do this for very long, just enough time to help with bringing about the awareness.

- Ask yourself what is going through the mind as you are experiencing the emotion. You may, in fact, be reacting to something else. Is the feeling yours? Are you taking on board someone else's emotions?

- Take a moment to 'feel' the emotion as if you are lying on a raft and floating through the emotion. Does it feel calm or brash? Soft or hard? Loud or quiet? Identify how the emotion feels by imagining the emotion or imagining yourself inside the emotion.

- Adjust the emotion. Just imagine you can see, hear and/or feel the dial and have the ability to turn the emotion up and/or down. You may once again use the idea of a **remote control**. Ask yourself how severe the emotion is, from one to ten, and if the emotion is a ten, ask yourself what you need to do to turn the dial back down to a lower number.

- Reconnect with the body. Placing the focus back onto the body helps you process the emotion. Feel the feet against the floor and let the shoulders drop. Just observe how it feels not to resist the force of gravity.

Chapter 5
Eating and Your Emotions

- Do not fight the feelings. The more you resist, the bigger the emotions and the feelings become because what you resist persists. Like a craving, those little voices persist and they will continue until you do something to acknowledge them and address the issue for which they are sending the message.

- Ask yourself if there is a positive intent of the emotion? Maybe you need to feel sadness or anger at this moment. Maybe you need to cry. Give yourself a few moments in which to do so and then let it go. Moving through the emotion and validating the emotion is a worthwhile experience and can help you better deal with the emotions. Allow yourself the time that you need to process your emotions. We all have many different parts which make up our personality and those parts have emotions. Your emotions can help you through difficult situations and it is healthy to express emotions in a positive manner.

- Do not punish yourself. Experience the emotion with a sense of compassion. If the emotion does not fit the situation, then this is a strong clue that part of you may need some assistance to heal a past hurt or trauma. This is a perfect example of where a therapy such as ego state therapy could be of assistance to you.

- You can also engage in a daily ritual like journaling, singing, saying a prayer or even meditating, depending on your own internal belief system, to better work through emotions.

Food addictions

> Food can be just as addictive as some drugs.
> Is food your drug of choice?

A recent study originally published in *The American Journal of Clinical Nutrition* suggests that certain types of foods can actually trigger addictive behaviours similar to addictive drugs. Drugs such as nicotine and cocaine, for example, rewire the brain so that it craves that 'high'. The desire is often so strong that it takes over all reasoning, as it becomes an all-consuming mission (Sifferlin, 2013).

MRI scans of obese men who participated in the study found that milkshakes consumed with higher glycaemic index levels (high GI) activated what is called the 'nucleus accumbens' which is the same trigger that aggravates the neurotransmitters with addictive drugs and alcohol. The study inferred that there was a connection between food and dependence in the fact that obese individuals may actually lose their sensitivity to leptin, which is a hormone that regulates hunger released by fat cells in the body (Sifferlin, 2013).

Nancy Appleton, PhD, in her book *Suicide by Sugar* infers that sugar can actually ruin health and suppress the immune system and that it can reduce the body's ability to defend itself against bacterial infection (Appleton, PhD & Jacobs, 2009).

> Too much sugar converts to fat causing obesity and poor teeth and premature aging (Appleton, PhD & Jacobs, 2009).

Appleton states 143 reasons why sugar ruins the health and looks at sugar as a highly addictive substance just like drugs or alcohol. Most of us do not view something like sugar as a drug, however, her research implies otherwise.

Addictions, whether they are food or drugs, all work in a similar fashion according to Appleton (2009). For example, drugs, including sugar, create dependencies in the brain; without these substances the levels of serotonin, which is a powerful neurotransmitter, drop. All addictive substances once consumed typically raise the serotonin levels for a short time resulting in a good feeling. The problem is, that feeling does not last and after the effects wear off, the serotonin levels drop rapidly and in some cases to a level even lower than prior to taking the substance.

This leaves the consumer feeling as if they have 'crashed'. Low levels of serotonin can even leave you feeling down or experiencing symptoms of depression. When the brain experiences these 'down' feelings it serves as a signal that it wants more of the addictive substance. The brain then sends messages to other neurotransmitters of the brain saying 'time to top up', so we can experience that good feeling once again. The problem is, over time it takes more and more of the addictive substance to experience the same 'high' and/or good feeling.

Another powerful neurotransmitter called 'dopamine' also plays a role in sugar addiction. Dopamine activates the brain's reward centre causing you to crave sweets even if you are not truly hungry. Take, for example, the idea of a piece of chocolate cake. If you happen to have a sweet tooth then you may become excited even thinking about a piece of chocolate cake. You can thank the brain's reward centre for this. When you eat the cake, the brain's reward centre is immediately activated, leaving you feeling happy. This tricks you into thinking that the chocolate cake actually makes you physically happy for a short time. However, this is not really the case – what is actually occurring is the sugar addiction tricks the brain (Gray, 2003).

Gray also talks about dopamine and serotonin in his book *The Mars and Venus Diet and Exercise Solution*, inferring that dopamine gives you energy and motivation while serotonin helps you relax (Gray, 2003). Gray's theory is that men and women process amino acids they eat in protein very differently, with men often having a dopamine deficiency and women having a serotonin deficiency (2003). Gray continues by stating that because of this, men tend to seek out behaviours that stimulate dopamine, like sports and action movies, while women, on the other hand, may seek the comfort and security of relationships because that tends to stimulate serotonin (Gray, 2003).

Cas, with her long-time experience of working within the field of various types of addictions, believes there is a direct correlation between the feelings and the emotions that have been interrupted by either an overload or an insufficient amount of serotonin and/or dopamine, which can erratically disturb the parts within a person's mind, resulting in internal conflict or trauma. Cas has found that addictive behaviours specifically focusing on food are almost always linked to the childhood developmental years, where the various parts have developed coping behaviours in an attempt to obtain the basic human needs of power, security, love, belonging, freedom, and fun. Cas has found that people can experience bouts of depression, stress, anxiety or fear which can lead to dysfunctional behaviours that may have a dramatic impact on a person's ability to function effectively in their day-to-day lives. This can be difficult to identify for the individual who may be experiencing the unhelpful behaviours and patterns. Often in order to ascertain the changes required, the assistance of a therapist may be needed.

These are some very interesting theories that you may wish to explore. In our opinion, what this really reveals is that food can be addictive. However, that does not mean that you are powerless to fight it because the mind is very powerful and by having awareness of it, you will be armed with the tools needed to overcome this and in fact many addictions.

NLP exercises to practise

We have included Neuro-Linguistic Programming (NLP) because we felt that this part of the process is assisted with the reprogramming that is required to ensure permanent change. NLP's basic premise is that we all perceive things a little differently depending on the experiences we have had throughout our lives.

John Grinder and Richard Bandler (1975) developed the premise behind NLP and theorised that the brain can actually learn healthier patterns and better ways of thinking that could bring about positive effects. We as humans have receptor systems, our five senses, which are sight, hearing, touch, taste and smell (Bandler & Grinder, 1975, p. 8). According to Bandler and Grinder (1975), we learn how to tap into those senses so that we can program our mind and body to respond accordingly. Often

Chapter 5
Eating and Your Emotions

the programming of the mind and body may need refining, which can occur through NLP techniques.

Each of us creates our own unique reality and our own internal map of the world through our previous and current programming and perceptions. You might be wondering what all of this has to do with weight management, bear with us, as we explain it has a lot to do with it.

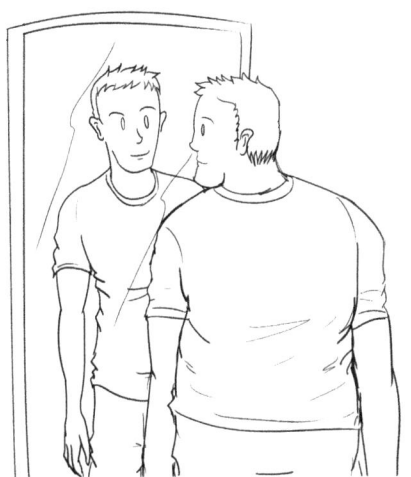

NLP uses the senses, using the mind to help you 'do different' and change behaviours. You can use the sense of sight, for example, and practise imagining yourself as a healthier, leaner person. Just close your eyes and take a few cleansing breaths, and then take a few moments to really see yourself as you wish to be. See yourself eating healthy meals, laughing with friends, feeling free to be you. See yourself wearing smaller clothes, feeling confident in your new body and feeling proud of yourself. Envision what kinds of choices you now make as a healthier, leaner person and envision how this changes your life.

Use the sense of touch to do the same, as you practise feeling the new healthier and leaner body. Imagine yourself running your hands up and down the body, really appreciating and respecting the body.

Use the sense of taste and imagine yourself taking small delectable bites of delicious healthy foods. Notice the refreshing tastes and how clean the mouth feels without a fatty residue.

Utilise your sense of smell, close your eyes and notice the aromas around you, absorb them, embracing a whole new appreciation of your relationship with food. Remember to tap into your hearing and listen to the sounds that stem from different foods when you are eating, chewing or even sucking, build upon your understanding of food and how it is absorbed into the body.

When you experience, even in the mind, how it feels to be healthy and vibrant, the subconscious mind takes in that feeling and it can manifest those feelings into reality.

Schedule some time each day to simply spend a few moments in silent reflection or meditation, seeing, feeling and tasting what it feels like to live in this new way, be surprised at how quickly and easily things start to change.

ACTIVITY 12: IMPORTANT NLP STEP

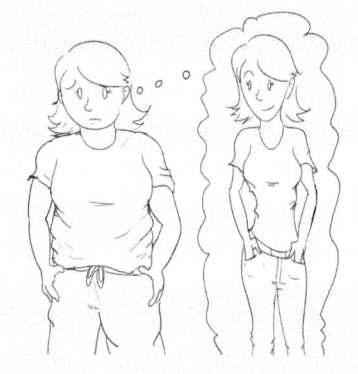

Buy something new, in the shape and size you want to be, the shape and size that IS right and healthy for you. It needs to be in the size that you want to be at your goal weight (you can do this in steps if you need, especially if the transformation is a big difference, and it can be of assistance to be imagined in steps.) This item must be something new with the store tags still attached to it and it cannot be something that you have worn before and wish to grow back into. There are memories and occasions associated with old items of clothing if you have worn them so it must be something that you have never worn. If you have clothing in your wardrobe and it still has the store tags attached and you have never worn it and there are no memories associated with the item, then that is okay.

Chapter 5
Eating and Your Emotions

When you have the selected clothing, you need to hang it in a prime position in your bedroom, perhaps over the wardrobe door, over the window or somewhere you are going to see it every morning when you wake up and every night before you sleep. Allow yourself to imagine being that size, enjoying being in that outfit. Imagine being in that item of clothing and enjoying every moment. Notice where you are and who you are with. It may be a specific occasion. Notice yourself being comfortable in that situation, make it fun and enjoyable. Really see it, feel it, hear it and be it. Live it and make it your reality.

The imagination is very powerful and wins every time. For example, let's say you are scared of heights. Now imagine we have a board about 150 mm or 6 inches wide and 50 metres long. If we lay that board down on the street and ask you to walk along that board, you would more than likely have no problem in doing so at all. Then if we take that exact same board and place it between two city buildings on about the twelfth floor, there is possibly no way that most people would even consider stepping out onto the board. This is because the imagination will be running wild with a lot of 'what ifs': 'What if I fall?', 'What if the board breaks?', 'What if a gust of wind blows unexpectedly?' The hands may begin to sweat, the legs may begin to shake, the stomach may begin to churn etc. and this is all simply by utilising the power of the mind and the imagination, hence, the reason behind why we want you to tap into that power and use the imagination to your benefit.

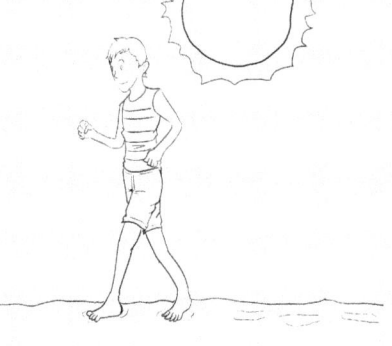

Imagine that you look sexy and great. Imagine yourself being exactly the shape and size you want to be. Just imagine having lots of fun, enjoying life and feeling good. Make sure you make it colourful and bright and give it sound. Give it everything that creates that bright strong powerful image. See it, hear it and feel it – you as the shape and size that is right and healthy for you. Really imagine it and give it all the possible energy that you can to make it your reality.

Imagine you are in it, living it, doing it, breathing it and imagine this every day, with passion and conviction. The more passionately you can imagine this, the more powerful the focus point is and the more powerful the pathway to your destination grows each day in every way.

To download an mp3 of Cas' positive affirmations go to:

www.CasWillow.com/HeyHeyAffirmations

and follow the instructions.

Chapter 6

The Role of Nutrition in Health

The ABCs of good nutrition

> A journey of a thousand miles begins with a single step
> (Lao-tzu).

As we venture into this process of weight management, the important focus to begin with is a discussion about good nutrition. Since this program is all about 'eating healthy, feeling healthy, thinking healthy, being healthy and living healthy', proper nutrition is most certainly a part of that process. What we place into our bodies makes a difference to how far it can run!

Poor nutrition can lead to poor health because poor nutrition can increase the risk factors for things like cardiovascular disease, high cholesterol, high blood pressure, heart disease, type 2 diabetes and even cancer and osteoarthritis. Childhood obesity has more than tripled over the last 30 years, which is a sad fact indeed. Obesity affects much more than just health; it also affects one's confidence and self-esteem.

The fact is that over a lifetime you will consume nearly 70,000 meals and over 60 tons of food (Fahey, Insel, & Roth, 2010). That is equivalent to nearly six solid years of eating! When you consider how much food the body will consume over a lifetime, proper nutrition is of integral importance. When it comes right down to it, what you eat really does affect your energy levels and your overall quality of health on a day-to-day basis.

Nutrition is the science that links foods to health and disease. It also includes the processes by which the body digests, absorbs, metabolises and excretes food. Real foods, which means foods that are fresh and unprocessed, provides the body with the proper energy that it needs to live a healthy lifestyle and also provides the body with energy to build and maintain the body's cells. When people eat processed foods their body struggles to sift through the toxins and work through what is left to allocate to the areas of the body that need the energy and strength.

Good nutrition is all about learning how to eat the foods that keep the body lean, vibrant and healthy, without going overboard in any one particular area. You are what you eat, so the food choices you make influence how you look and feel.

When you eat lean, healthy, fresh and unprocessed foods, the body thrives and when you eat foods that do not support the body, the body holds on to extra weight as a result.

The truth is that you can never gain from supplements and processed foods what Mother Nature herself can provide through proper nutrition. Most of the vitamins and minerals you need to achieve and maintain optimal health can be found by eating real foods, fresh from nature.

Incorporating real foods into your diet is easier than you might think. Shopping in the organic produce section and the lean protein section can go a long way to helping you achieve and maintain a healthy way of eating. It is never too late to start a healthy eating regime because every choice you make today helps you live better tomorrow.

> The goal of proper nutrition in this program is 'balanced, healthy moderation and awareness of the body'.

Most people know what they need to eat to keep the body healthy. The goal of nutrition in this program is 'balanced, healthy moderation and awareness of the body'. If you feel sick after eating a particular food, then you might want to reconsider eating that food in the future. The body is your best indicator of what is healthy and nutritious for you. If you eat a particular food and feel great, then the body is giving you a clear signal that you have eaten a healthy food that is right for you.

The subconscious mind knows what type of food is right and healthy for you and what type of food is consistent with good health and good weight management. You know how to eat healthy, so from this moment forward it is simply a matter of making better choices, choices that support a healthy body and a healthy mind.

When you make a commitment to eat to live, you can choose to eat foods that are in alignment with your weight management goals. You have the power to choose what you place into your mouth so that you feel refuelled and ready to engage with the world.

Healthy nutritious foods are good for the body and good for the brain. When you aim for a well-balanced healthy eating plan you are making a smart choice. The best plan is one that is 'Back to the Basics' and easy to live with each day of your life.

Planting the seeds

> Just as you plant seeds in a garden, you also plant seeds within the mind.

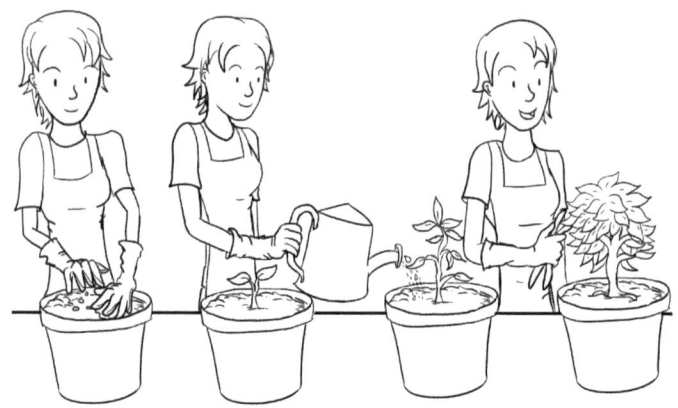

The process of living healthy and being healthy is like planting a seed in many ways. When you plant a seed in a garden you are well aware that seeds take time to grow. Seeds need to be watered, tended to and cared for. If you ignore the seed it will fail to thrive. If you water the seed and send it love on a regular basis, the seed rewards you by growing. Just as a garden is not created overnight, the process of obtaining optimum health for each individual person takes a little time. By focusing on the state of health you are aiming for you can more easily attain that state of health. You are important; you are what matters; you are your own authority of your mind and you are the only one who can control you, no one else.

Just as you plant seeds in a garden you also plant seeds in the mind. The truth is that seeds planted within the mind can form and create thoughts which you can choose to become your reality. Deliberately planting conscious thoughts in the mind can assist with the creation of a different reality of your choice.

Affirmations are a wonderful way to plant seeds in the mind. Affirmations, as the name implies, affirm that which you believe to be true or that which you would like to be true. The mind takes things very literally and that is why some self-talk is so damaging. Affirmations of empowerment as a focus point can help you create the state of mind or the state of health that you are looking to produce.

Many times our words work against us. We say things to ourselves that are damaging or hurtful. Even something silly like 'Wow, why did I do that, that was really dumb' can send the wrong message to the mind. The mind is a reflection of thoughts and thoughts create reality. When you affirm that you are lean, healthy and vibrant, the mind takes a hold of that statement as if it were already true and, before you know it, you become that which you affirm or think.

It is important to give your subconscious mind crisp, clear and clean language that it understands, because the subconscious mind does NOT analyse the overall sentence it hears. It takes each word as it has been programmed to understand the meaning of that word. For example, if you were asked 'How are you feeling today?' and let's say you are neither good nor bad, so you reply 'Not too bad'. In everyday language we could analyse this to mean 'Pretty good' or average, not on a high or a low. The choice you make here, whilst not important on a conscious level, is vital on a subconscious level. If you say 'Not too bad', the subconscious mind, which does not analyse, hears 'I am bad' – so why not simply develop the habit of flipping from the negative to the positive response of 'Pretty good' so the subconscious mind hears 'I am good'. Another example would be 'Don't think of a pink elephant'. Your subconscious mind now has an image of a pink elephant due to the fact that the subconscious mind did not analyse the entire sentence, which said *don't* think of it. Did you also notice that the elephant you imagined was pink? If you analyse that with the logic of your conscious mind you will also know that real life elephants are not pink. However, with the power of the mind you can imagine anything you wish to be your reality.

Feeling worthy of good things in life is important for your happiness and your health. When you feel worthy, you feel like you deserve good things. Feeling worthy means to feel confident and deserving. It is about knowing and realising that you deserve to be happy, fit and healthy and there is no better time like the present in which to begin this process.

When you eliminate negative mindsets and destructive patterns, the garden of the mind prospers and thrives.

When you affirm something, you plant a tiny little seed in the mind. When the mind hears a positive statement repeated day in and day out, it believes that statement to be true and manifests it into your life. You can think of affirmations as gentle little reminders of the life you have and desire. This process you are about to undertake is akin to pulling the weeds in the garden. When you eliminate adverse mindsets and destructive patterns, the garden of the mind prospers and thrives. You replace self-doubt with helpful thoughts and those thoughts create your new reality.

This process is all about thinking differently and thinking in terms of vitality and good health. When you affirm that you are 'eating healthy, feeling healthy, thinking healthy, being healthy and living healthy', you plant new seeds and create a fertile environment for those seeds to grow.

Learning how to eat REAL nourishing food

This process is not about deprivation, as the definition of deprivation is to not have enough and this is not just about food. This is also about having fun, having freedom, having security, having protection, and belonging, which are all of our basic human needs. These needs, including eating healthy and loving the body, must be met.

In the end, remember that food is merely fuel because nothing tastes quite as good as sexy feels. You can still enjoy food, just like you did before, just in smaller more reasonable amounts. When you really take the time to appreciate your food and become mindful of your food, you begin to look at food a little differently.

Chapter 6
The Role of Nutrition in Health

When you program into the mind thoughts that you are easily satisfied with just a small amount of food, the mind then makes it so. The practice of mindful eating is a wonderful practise because it allows you to really enjoy your food.

When you can learn to slow down the process of eating, it becomes a much more enjoyable process. When you start exercising and moving the body the mind releases powerful chemical endorphins, which make you literally feel better. When you feel better, you treat the body much more respectfully. This process is really about love – loving the body and loving the mind. It is important to appreciate the parts of the body and the role that each part plays in the effective functioning of the body. For example, the feet are precious and assist us to stand and walk, and our hands write, clap, hold and direct us. It is only when our ability to use certain parts of the body is taken away from us, that we realise the importance of those parts and how much we have taken our bodies for granted. It is about treating yourself with the love and the respect you so deserve.

> This process is really about love – loving
> the body and loving the mind.

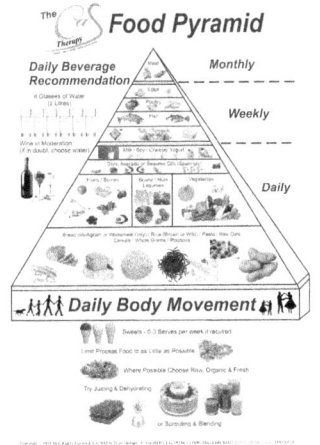

Eating real food is really quite a simple process. Processed foods typically have much of the nutritional value 'processed' out. If you can commit to making a few small changes over time, the process becomes much simpler. Here are a few tips to transitioning to eating real nourishing foods. You can use the 'Food Pyramid' to help you with choices.

(There is a larger Food Pyramid on page 121).

To download the Food Pyramid pdf simply go to: www.CasWillow.com/castherapyfoodpyramid.pdf

Hey Hey It's Me!

Tips for eating real nourishing foods

- Eat more REAL carbohydrates and less processed foods.
    - This is such an important step because many processed foods are devoid of nutritional value. Although it may be a little challenging at first, once you become more accustomed to eating real foods like fresh fruits and vegetables, it easily becomes a lifelong eating pattern.

- Eat more lean proteins.
    - By choosing a variety of lean, healthy proteins like organic and grass-fed meat, tofu, eggs and free-range chicken and other types of lean proteins you can actually increase your metabolism by up to 30%. When you eat protein you also feel more satisfied.

- Eat healthy fats.
    - This includes olive oil, coconut oil, avocados, seeds and nuts.

- Experiment with greens.
    - There are so many choices when it comes to healthy greens. Try some kale chips for a pleasant change or look online for recipes for foods you would not usually choose.
    - For a complimentary sample of some simple Tasty Vegan Recipes, go to www.HealthyVeganLiving.com and enter your name and email address.

ACTIVITY 13: EATING IN A HEALTHY MANNER
More tips for eating in a healthy manner

- Choose smaller plates – this is so the mind is not seeing a small amount on a large plate which can provoke feelings of deprivation. This is very effective and becomes satisfying for the mind and the body.

- STOP – check for the full and satisfied signals and messages being sent by the stomach. Do not use the mind as an indicator; listen to the signals and messages from the body.
- Watch your portions – always check for proper serving sizes. Many of us are eating 2–3 times above what is considered a normal serving size, purely from habit. Our bodies only need small amounts of food to function efficiently. Did you know that our stomachs are approximately the same size as a clenched fist?

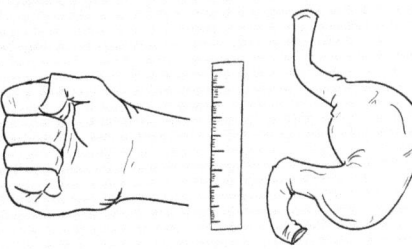

- Drink more water and less soft drinks.
- Skip the fancy coffee – it has a lot of hidden sugars and fats.
- Steer away from fried foods and go for baked or grilled.
- Clear away junk food from your kitchen.
- Pack healthy snacks and take them with you when you are on the go.
- Dine out less often.
- Order your salad dressing on the side.
- Shop at your local farmers market and experiment with local foods.
- Skip the dessert and order fresh fruit.
- Eat smaller, more frequent meals – this keeps the body replenished.
- Never skip meals – starving the body triggers the deprivation part of you and the body will begin to slow the metabolism believing

it is not receiving any food. Our ancestors trained our bodies to instinctively store fats as they were either subject to a feast or a famine, and were unsure of their next meal. Unfortunately, in Western society our famine only lasts as long as it takes us to drive to the local supermarket and this is just not healthy for living a balanced life.

- Seek out organic and nourishing, or home grown, foods.
- If you feel stressed or anxious, notice that part of you and thank that part and then take a nice long walk instead of reaching for a snack. Stop looking to fill empty. Empty is okay with being empty or sometimes even half empty.

Eating healthy is not complicated. In fact eating healthy is really a lifestyle choice, a choice that helps the body prosper and thrive in an energetic manner. Eating healthy is only a part of the full living healthy lifestyle pathway. Living the lifestyle that creates energy, motivation, excitement and stimulation comes from the holistic approach. Refer back to the 'Living a Healthy Lifestyle Circle' on page 90 to keep you on track.

> The secret of success is to be in harmony with existence,
> to be always calm, to let each wave of life wash us
> a little farther up the shore (Barnett, 2006).

Living and eating healthy as a lifestyle choice

It has been proven time and time again that living a healthy lifestyle is important in terms of preventing chronic disease. It is really quite simple to live a healthy lifestyle, and it is more of an attitude than anything else.

> Eating healthy is a lifestyle choice – it is
> a mindset and a philosophy.

Chapter 6
The Role of Nutrition in Health

You really do not have to change that much when you make that commitment to live in a healthy manner. You do not have to become a vegetarian or eat raw foods unless of course that is your choice. You can take steps to avoid toxins in foods by simply choosing fresh fruits and whole vegetables. You can make the choice to take a brisk walk 3–4 times a week. You can stop smoking if you currently smoke, and you can make a conscious effort to be respectful of the body. After all, the body is your vehicle to carry you through this lifetime. Therefore, you need to nurture it, look after and maintain your vehicle daily, just like you need to maintain your car and give it the correct fuel if you wish it to run effectively and efficiently.

The modern lifestyle is certainly convenient, however, it can also be very unhealthy. The choices you make today really do impact the life you will live tomorrow, so every small choice you make towards greater health makes a big long-term difference.

When you start eating and living in a healthier manner, the body thrives. You feel better, you look better and you rarely become sick. Eating healthy is a lifestyle choice. It becomes a mindset and a philosophy. When you trust this process and have faith in yourself, you form a solid foundation.

This process is really about learning to eat to refuel the body, moving away from emotional eating and moving towards a healthier lifestyle.

Learning what the body needs for vibrant health and learning to read the body's signals are key principles towards living a healthy lifestyle.

How do you know when you are truly hungry or if you are merely eating out of habit? Sometimes we overeat for other reasons besides hunger. Learning to recognise the body's hunger signals is an important part of this process.

> Taking a step back, returning to the basic human programming of the mind, living a healthy lifestyle, and managing your weight, is an everyday occurrence.

Often we make the process of weight management too complicated. Taking a step back, returning to the basic human programming of the mind, living a healthy lifestyle, and managing your weight, is an everyday occurrence. When you develop an effective mental attitude and you really want to gain improved health, you can use that emotion and that passion to shift your thinking and to change your behaviour. If you really and truly want this to happen, then it WILL happen because you WILL make it happen.

Understanding your own motivation and eating habits is an extremely valuable weight management tool. While appetite is psychological and hunger is physiological, often it is difficult to tell the difference between the messages.

Researchers have been studying the various influences that play a role in appetite versus hunger for many years. The body is increasingly complex. Things called hunger hormones or ghrelin that exist in the blood and in the empty stomach work together to signal to the brain that you are hungry.

Nerves in the brain also send signals that you are full, however, those signals can take up to 20 minutes to go through – and by that time, you may have already eaten too much.

The old adage that it takes 20 minutes to realise you are full is actually quite true, so eating more slowly is one thing you can do, as it allows more time for that signal to arrive. If you spend longer than 20 minutes eating, which is certainly recommended, you may actually find that you are sufficiently full, even before you push away from the table.

When you can learn to stop before you are really comfortably full, you give the mind and the body time to process the food you have just consumed. Remember, the importance of being cognisant of the body's signals. The more you increase your awareness and become in tune with your body, the easier this process is and the healthier you will become. The mind and body need to feel satisfied, not necessarily full, just satisfied. The important aspect about feeling satisfied is that you create that feeling and belief that you are satisfied.

Stop for a moment and observe what we may often find ourselves saying prior to a meal. You may find yourself saying something like 'I'm starving', 'I'm hungry', or 'I could eat a horse'. Notice then how the language and message to yourself changes between your main meal and sweets. You now may find yourself saying something like 'I think I can fit that in' or 'That looks nice'. Notice how before sweets the message may be interpreted that you are no longer hungry in the stomach, therefore no longer hungry for food, leaving us with the question: 'What are you really hungry for?' Clearly it is no longer food.

Tips for handling hunger

- Enjoy everything – in moderation. This is one of the keys to keeping this process simple. When you live a healthy lifestyle you realise you do not have to deprive yourself. You can enjoy all those foods you love, as long as you only eat a small bite or two and stop before you become too full.
- Remember, the eyes are always bigger than the stomach – the more food you put on your plate, the more you will eat!
- Eat foods that have volume like soups, hot cereals and cooked whole grains.
- Remember the fibre. Foods high in fibre like vegetables, fruits, legumes and even popcorn, are always smarter choices that help the digestive system.
- Steer clear of the buffet line. You might tend to eat more.
- Snack on lean protein, including tofu and dates.

- Remember, when you select the food and pick the food up to eat, ask:
    - What will this food do for me?
    - Will it give me energy?
    - Will it make me sleep?
    - Will it affect my mood?

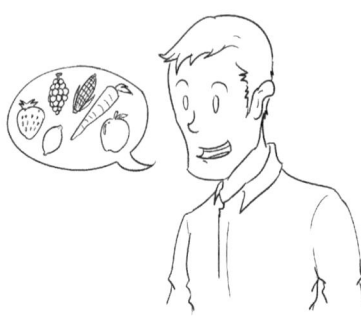

Everything we eat does something to us or for us. It is important to recognise what is in the best interests and health for our body.

You are what you eat, so the healthier you eat and the more respect you treat the body with, the better off you will be at the end of the day. As we have stated before, this process is not about deprivation; it is about healthy living. When you really begin to take hold of this concept, you begin 'eating healthy, feeling healthy, thinking healthy, being healthy and living healthy' and that is what this book is ALL about.

> If you really and truly want this to happen, then it WILL happen because you WILL make it happen.

ACTIVITY 14: FOOD PYRAMID

Notice and plan your Food Pyramid with your daily body movement.

As mentioned earlier in this chapter, to download a full colour pdf copy of the CaS Therapy Food Pyramid with our compliments visit: www.CasWillow.com/castherapyfoodpyramid.pdf

Chapter 6
The Role of Nutrition in Health

The CaS Food Pyramid

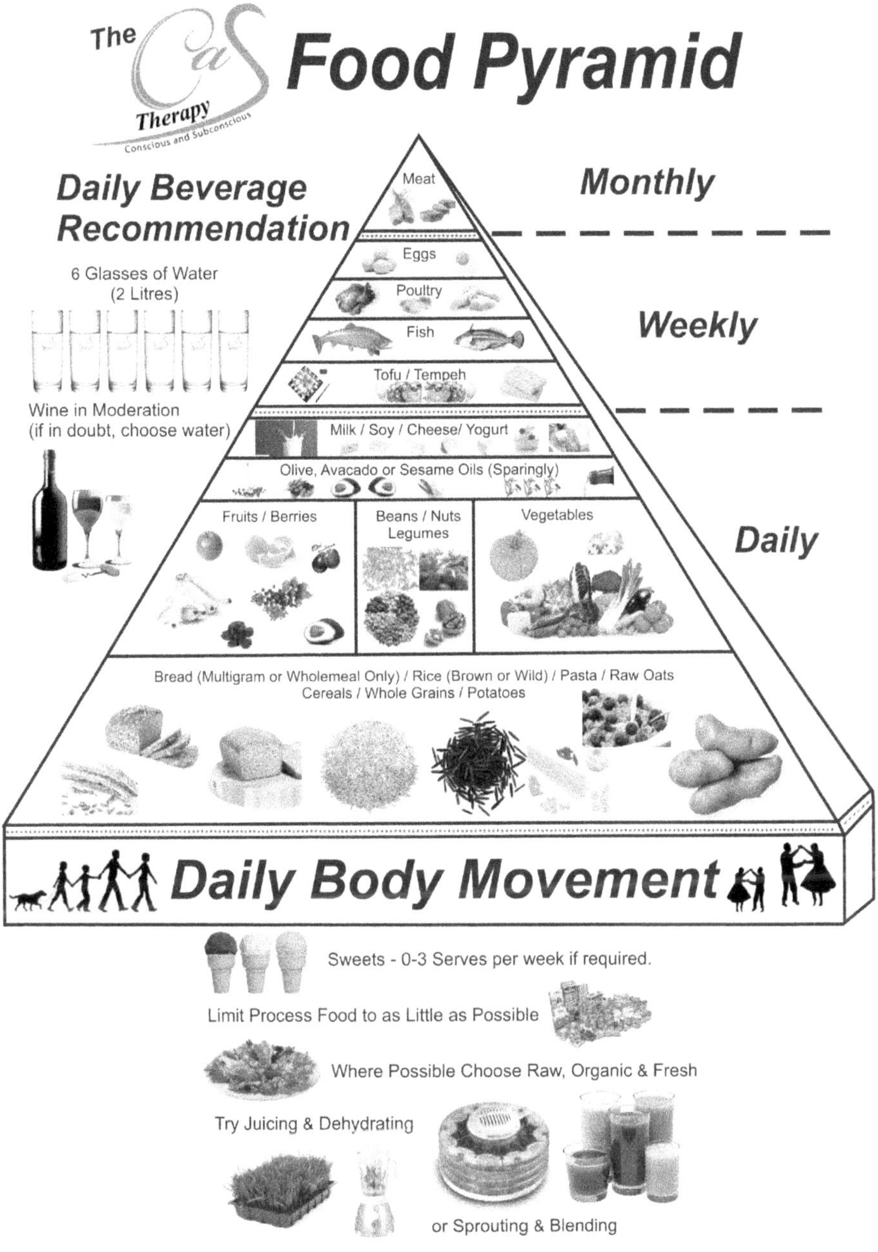

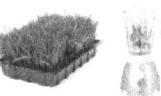

Chapter 7

The Clean Slate Process

Identifying limiting beliefs that serve no purpose

> Cleaning the slate is the key to the transformation process.
> It allows you to reprogram the subconscious mind
> with healthy patterns of behaviour and mindsets.

What kind of beliefs do you hold when it comes to weight management? What has worked for you and what has not worked? Do you think it is difficult to manage your weight? Have you 'tried' every 'diet' under the sun? Do you feel as if you have a slow metabolism? Do you find it challenging to stick to a healthy eating plan? Do your cravings drive you crazy?

There are many reasons why you may believe it is all too hard. We are often analysing our thought processes because our thoughts guide us in many ways. If you were always told you were a 'big eater' then subconsciously you may still believe that.

If someone said something harsh to you as a child like, 'You will always be fat', then part of you may still believe that, even though you are an adult. Yes, that part of you which was formed in your developmental years as a child may still believe that to be true, therefore, that part acts accordingly. Thoughts consume us and thoughts can rule us if we jump into our thoughts and ride them. For example, Cas truly believed in her early adulthood that she would be 'big' for the rest of her life, like she had been programmed to believe throughout her childhood by her family. It was not until she researched how the mind worked that she challenged her childhood belief system. When you start to analyse and unpack layers of beliefs that serve no helpful purpose, you clear the way to begin the process of moving forward.

This process you are undergoing allows you to gently shift the mindset from thoughts of 'not good enough' and possible feelings of deprivation to thoughts that bring about vibrant health and feelings that match the way of life you choose.

As we have seen, excess weight can sometimes be a mask for other emotional conditions. Our beliefs are self-perpetuating in many ways, because thoughts can become obstacles that have the ability to block your growth and development.

Cleaning the slate is the key transformation process. It allows you to reprogram the subconscious mind and program the conscious part of the mind with more healthy behaviours and mindsets.

The cleaning the slate process utilises the **FLiPiT** method. We focus on **Freeing** the old words that keep people stuck, and then **Lift** ourselves with new meaningful words **Increasing** the power of those **Positive** words to oneself. Next we **Include** the reinforcement of a person's real truths which **Transforms** anything and everything into what the person wants and desires.

FLiPiT, as discussed in the 7 Life Steps, can be utilised throughout any area of life to bring about change.

Chapter 7
The Clean Slate Process

> # FLIPIT
>
> * F – Free – The Old Words
> * L – Lift – The New Words
> * I – Increase – The meaning of the words
> * P – Positive – Reinforcement
> * I – Include – Real truths
> * T – Transform – anything & everything

This process identifies the threads that tie unhelpful behaviours to the past, which then allows you to release them so they do not impact on you in the now and in the future. You see, when we carry our hurtful and painful thoughts, feelings, difficult memories, personal experiences, self-torture attitudes, even secrets, we can become tired and exhausted with the constant struggle. Often what we carry can become an obstacle, specifically if it sits right in front of a person wanting to move forward. This obstacle blocks the pathway to connect and engage with life. In order to remove the obstacles we need to disconnect or simply make room for the emotion from that experience and allow the experiences to be in their own space within the past. Remember that we need to manage our emotions and painful experiences, not ignore them or store them, so you can then engage and connect more freely with life. Cleaning the slate is about keeping the memories, the learnings and the experiences and simply releasing all that stops you from moving forward. The important factor here is to ensure that we make room for all that is you, so release the threads that pull you back and keep you 'stuck'.

What is it you believe when it comes to weight management?

Activity 15: Underlying Associations

Take a moment now and think about all of those underlying associations you have when it comes to maintaining a healthy weight:

- Being fat is genetic.
- Diets are difficult.
- Eating healthy takes too much work.
- I will always be big because my family is big.
- I have no idea how to eat healthy.
- I will just fail again.
- I don't like starving myself.
- Exercise is hard and I don't have enough time.
- Diets are depressing.
- I like food too much to give anything up.
- Food makes me feel better.
- Food is love and comfort.
- I have always had trouble losing weight.
- I don't have enough energy to exercise.
- I am too busy to cook.
- I feel embarrassed going to a health club.
- I don't feel good about myself.

- I am just not motivated.
- I have tried diets and they don't work for me.
- I am not good enough to have a good body.
- I am ugly, so I will always be ugly, even when I am thin.
- It's all too hard.

To how many did you identify with and say 'Yes, that's me too'?

How often do we allow these underlying beliefs to stop us from becoming the shape and size that is right and healthy for us and living the healthy lifestyle we choose?

Are you going to let these beliefs stop you from moving forward? 'Yes' or 'no'? STOP and take the time to think and analyse your answer to this question. This is the time to answer truthfully. If your answer is 'no' then go back to Step 3.

What is the belief behind this?

Sometimes we can be our own worst enemy. Simply put, we often stand in our own way. We criticise ourselves and put ourselves down. Why? Why would we sabotage ourselves when it comes to achieving a healthy weight? STOP and take a moment to ask yourself if there may be a secondary gain to staying at an unhealthy weight. As strange as this may seem, it does happen. Some people carry around excess weight as a shield of protection because they do not want to be noticed. It may be easier for them to repel attention and to then be socially invisible, rather than being noticed.

There are many possible reasons behind why people carry excess weight, some of which include programming beliefs, patterns and behaviours during the developmental years; other reasons could be more painful, physical, emotional and/or sexual abuse issues. Whatever

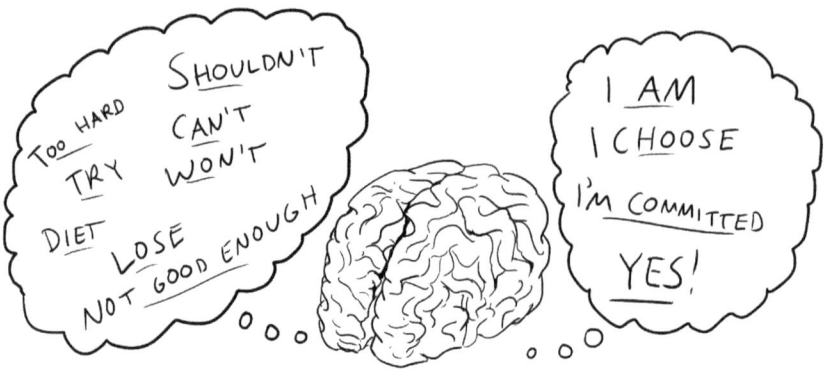

the initial cause, the weight is there for a reason and the parts of you that are continuing to overeat, make unhealthy choices and have minimal awareness, are protecting you and working with you in some way, sometimes in a way we would prefer they did not. However, all of the parts are on your side and they are of the belief that what they are doing is in your best interest. If you are aware of any abuse or trauma from your past, we highly recommend you seek the professional assistance from a qualified and registered therapist. Of course, if you are close to a CaS Therapy Centre, we would be honoured to assist you in a private, confidential, safe and secure setting. If you are not near CaS Therapy, then a simple internet search for your local national accredited association will be able to assist you, or if you would prefer, email our centre and we will be able to direct you to an association that will be able to supply you with an extensive list of qualified therapists in close proximity to you.

> Limiting beliefs are a lot like roadblocks in the mind. They are in the way and they need to be moved out of the way.

Weight management does not have to be a painful and negative process. It can be an easy, exciting and energising 'Weigh of Life' as you think yourself thin and live a healthy lifestyle, one where you are totally aware of and have insight to the reactions and responses of the mind and body.

Chapter 7
The Clean Slate Process

You are in control of your thoughts and you are the authority of your own mind. You have everything you need within your mind. Your mind is like a library full of tools, strategies and techniques, which, if you choose and discover how to, you can access at any given time. The mind has the ability to accept new thought processes and to manage and accept any difficult and/or painful feelings and emotions, coupled with the ability to develop new patterns of behaviour. The subconscious mind continues to collate all of your experiences, values, beliefs, training, and knowledge as we travel through our journey of life. With this understanding and knowledge, you can access anything the subconscious holds, so you can have the choice to alter and modify any thoughts, feelings and behaviours in the present to create your future. An important factor is to utilise what we have learnt in the past. However, it is equally important to understand that what has occurred in your past is just a memory or an image and you are not living that past now. Often we allow our past experiences to define who we are today by making decisions based on the past. Remember that our past is only a part of us, not all of us, therefore, we need to identify who we are today and who we want to be tomorrow.

Before you can create new thoughts and patterns of behaviour, it is important to identify the old ones so that you can further understand why you still find it necessary to carry them around.

Limiting beliefs are a lot like roadblocks in the mind. They are in the way and they need to be moved out of the way. Many emotional patterns are established in our childhood and are, in turn, burned into the subconscious mind where they are repeated in a never-ending dialogue, resulting in unwanted behaviours.

Some people can trace their unhealthy eating patterns to one specific event in their childhood, while others find other trigger points. Food is such a source of comfort for so many people and we are sure many of you can recall times in your childhood where someone gave you food and you felt better as a result. This is interpreted by the subconscious mind as a 'reward'. We often bring that 'reward' behaviour with us into adulthood because we still seek the same warm accepting feelings of approval and comfort, as this is a basic human need.

These types of associations can be very powerful and long lasting, and something as simple as someone giving you a biscuit or a cupcake when you fell and hurt yourself as a child, can cause you to associate food with love, caring and healing.

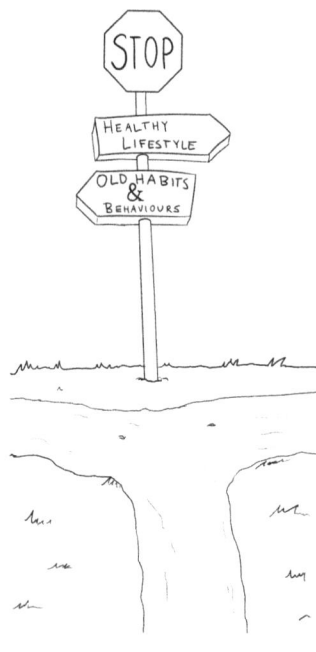

These types of memories can actually create emotional connections between food and comfort and you might subconsciously recall this every time you look at something sweet. Understanding the core of the issue can be quick, simple and easier than you may think. Part of reprogramming the mind is to help you choose fresh foods, like fruits and vegetables, to live, feel, be, think and eat healthy and to gain the motivation you need to exercise. There are many techniques, including hypnotherapy, that can help you say no to junk foods and unnecessary snacking and allow you to choose fresh unprocessed foods that the subconscious mind knows are conducive to better health and weight management that is natural and healthy for you.

An important factor to remember is that this process of programming has taken many years to develop. Certain mindsets and habits unique to you, based on your life experiences, can take time to discover and to reprogram a pathway that is suitable to you and your needs for your life journey.

> If you tell yourself every day that weight management is an easy and effortless process, then that is what it will be!

In the grand scheme of things, you are whatever you think you are. If you are constantly telling yourself that you have great difficulties managing your weight, then most likely as a result you will have great difficulties managing your weight.

On the other hand, if you tell yourself every day that weight management is easy and effortless for you, then as a result that is what it will be! This may sound way too simple, because it really is that simple. You need to make the decision to 'do different'. By making this decision you begin to trust and believe in the process and in turn you slowly begin to trust and believe in yourself.

Reasons that could be affecting your ability to manage your weight

ACTIVITY 16: LIST 10 REASONS

Let's ask YOU some simple questions when it comes to your beliefs about weight management. These could also be called the: who, what, when, where and why of weight management.

1. Why do you feel you cannot easily manage your weight?
2. What is keeping you from achieving your ideal shape and size?
3. When is the worst time of day for you when it comes to eating?
4. Who or what is keeping you from becoming and staying motivated?
5. Where do you eat most of your meals?
6. What is stopping you from exercising?
7. Are you afraid to become the shape and size you desire? If so, why?

8. What would it take for you to let the weight go?
9. What would life look like if you were your ideal shape and size?
10. How would your life be different?

Taking the time to answer these questions will be a step towards change and will help you gain the motivation you need to move forward. Once you identify your issues, or limiting beliefs, you can easily understand what might be holding you back.

Let's begin now and list 10 reasons in your journal, NIB or below why you might struggle with weight management. You can also look at these 'reasons' as your 'excuses' or your 'buts' if that makes it easier. However remember, nothing good ever comes in your life from a 'but'. Take your time, even come back to this later if you choose. Be as honest as you can with yourself, as this is your life and how you want to 'do different' begins with 'YOU'.

10 reasons why I believe weight management is difficult

1. _____

2. _____

3. _____

4. _____

5. _____

6. _____

7. _____

8. _____

9. _____

10. _____

Converting those reasons to positive statements

The next step involves converting those reasons to positive statements or affirmations. This is really quite simple to do. For example, if one of the reasons why you snack is that you do not have time to eat healthy, you could turn that statement around and phrase it something like: '*I always keep healthy snack items on hand when I am busy because I love healthy food.*'

Make sure these statements are set in the present tense, as if you have already achieved your goal. Living in the 'NOW' is the most important aspect to bringing about the change you want and desire. Being present lets the subconscious mind know that you are committed to living, being, thinking, feeling and eating healthy.

Another example would be if you feel you are unmotivated to exercise in the gym. You might rephrase that and say something like: '*I make time to exercise and move my body by finding different and unique ways to exercise outside of the gym.*'

You can see this is a relatively simple process. It is important to keep the suggestions in the present tense and ensure they are positive, because the mind will focus on whatever you tell it on a continual basis. If thoughts come into the mind that perhaps you find unhelpful, simply remember to allow the thoughts to be there in the mind; make room for those thoughts as they are important. You do not have to like or love those thoughts, however, you will find it helpful not to judge or criticise those thoughts. Just simply thank those thoughts, let them drift away, then invite and choose the thoughts you choose to give more energy to. Thanking those thoughts simply helps you to be more focused on the here and now which enhances your awareness of having thoughts. This helps you to focus on you, to actually think about what you are thinking about, which can only influence your current behaviours. When we think about what we are thinking about, the mind starts to look through different lenses, assisting with the interpretation process which brings about conscious awareness. This is called metacognition, thinking about thinking what you are thinking about, a normal process of the cognition of the mind.

Take a moment and do this now. Using statements that begin with 'I am', 'I feel' or 'I have', write them in your journal, NIB or below.

Chapter 7
The Clean Slate Process

ACTIVITY 17: 10 POSITIVE AFFIRMATIONS
10 positive affirmations for weight management

1. _____

2. _____

3. _____

4. _____

5. _____

6. _____

7. _____

8. _____

9. _____

10. _____

The clean slate exercise

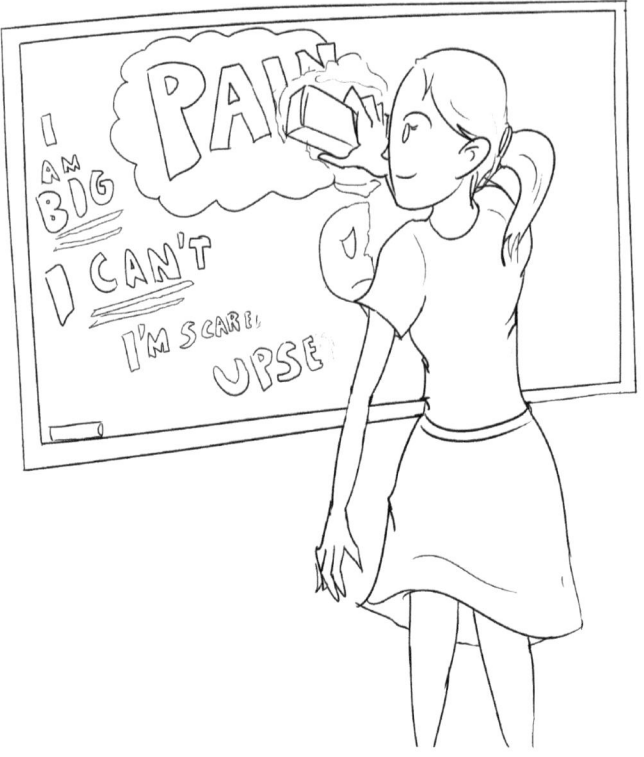

ACTIVITY 18: CLEAN SLATE

This exercise is designed to help you clean the slate, which will help you eliminate limiting beliefs and old mindsets, allowing you to start fresh. What we mean by 'cleaning the slate' is that after releasing old patterns and behaviours, we can keep the learnings from our past and then wipe away the old road map of our life that had no real direction and replace it with a road map that has a clear direction and focus.

Again, you may stop anywhere along the way to close your eyes and pause and reflect. You may choose to read each passage stopping

Chapter 7
The Clean Slate Process

to visualise the suggestions along the way, or you may read through the entire piece.

The clean slate

You may begin by taking a few deep and cleansing breaths. Just allow yourself to sink into relaxation and peace. Be one with the breath as it moves in and out of the body, becoming calmer and more relaxed with each breath.

Continue breathing in and out, until you feel a sense of peace, relaxation and calmness throughout the entire body. Take yourself to a beautiful, safe and comfortable place. Feel what you feel, see what you see and hear what you hear.

Now begin by visualising, or just have a sense or a feeling, of a large whiteboard right there in front of you. If you desire, you can envisage yourself at a lovely place like a beach or a park. Picture some place where you feel relaxed and at ease. Imagine in front of you is a large whiteboard on a mobile stand. The whiteboard has a duster, a cloth, textas, cleaning solution and a chisel, yes, a chisel, for anything that has become stuck and/or difficult to move. There is also a magic wand there, just in case.

Stop and Reflect...

As you reflect upon your life, start thinking about all of those things you associate with your weight management lifestyle struggle. You may choose to list things like:

- Yoyo dieting.
- Deprivation.
- Foods.
- Lack of enthusiasm.

- All of the emotional hurt and/or pain you have been through like sadness, depression, guilt, and disappointment.
- Obstacles or roadblocks.
- Can't have, shouldn't have, not supposed to have.
- Pictures or drawings you associate with this struggle.
- It's too hard.
- I can't lose weight.
- Social isolation.
- Feelings of insecurity.
- Unworthiness.
- Etc. etc. (anything that serves you no purpose).

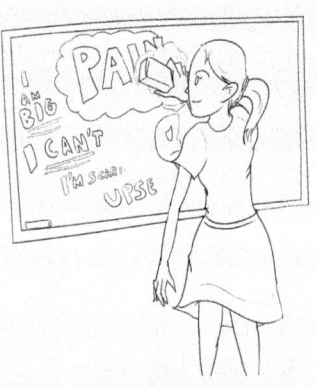

Write them, throw them or have them appear on that board, layer upon layer, covering and filling the entire board. You can write things several times, or just once, whatever you need. It is up to you as this is your time to free yourself so you can move forward.

Now take a look at what you have written on the board and ask yourself if this fully exemplifies your struggle when it comes to your weight and lifestyle. Just reflect and take a moment and see if anything else comes to mind. Now is the time to add to the board any symbols, numbers or colours that are floating through the mind, which are relevant to the cleansing process we are undertaking. It does not matter if things do not make sense on a conscious level.

Chapter 7
The Clean Slate Process

The next step is to look and reflect at the contents on the board and allow the subconscious part of the mind and the relevant parts of the mind to take and absorb any relevant learnings that appear before you. The intention here is to allow the parts to make the adjustments as the intention of all of our parts is always to benefit us in some way, sometimes in a way we would prefer they did not. However, all of the parts of us are offering some type of beneficial role. For example, if a part of you is experiencing stress, another part identifies that you feel calm and relaxed when you have a coffee and eat a chocolate cake, so that part's intention is to make you calm and relaxed. It does not realise the behaviour is not in your best interest with regard to living a healthy lifestyle.

Stop and Reflect...

Now let us slowly begin to clean the board. We will work from right to left so we can start fresh and go back in time. We are resetting your foundation and your program so we can start fresh. Now imagine a clean white cloth in your hand and start in the right hand corner wiping away and cleaning away the old mindsets and thought patterns, saying 'thank you mind, thank you parts, thank you body'. This is an important part of the process as we need to acknowledge that our past has served a purpose and is the reason we are where we are today.

Take as much time as you need to do this as there is no reason to rush. As you clean the board reflect upon what you can learn from examining the old ways of thinking.

Stop and Reflect...

You might notice some of the words and phrases wipe off quite easily while others leave an impression, even after you clean them. You may need to gather some more supplies to clean some of the more challenging behaviours away. Scrub as long as you need, use the cleaning solution, the chisel or even the magic wand if you need to.

If you need to, you may use another clean cloth and some cleaning spray so you can really erase all of the concepts and outdated patterns of thinking, so you can have a fresh, clean slate.

Stop and Reflect...

Now take one final look and notice if there are any imprints still left on the board. If so, what can you learn from them? Take one last clean sweep across the board and stand back and acknowledge and accept your efforts. You have now reclaimed your inner power and inner knowing ready to move forward in a new direction of your choice.

Stop and Reflect...

Now place a lacquer on the board so you can start fresh with new ideals and a new healthy mindset. Allow the lacquer to set, whilst you allow the body and mind to adjust and move through the transition of this change.

If you like, you may even choose to write a new phrase that now exemplifies your new way of thinking such as: '*I am living a healthy lifestyle and I always will. I eat healthy, I feel healthy and I think healthy.*'

Nicely done!

Your FREEDOM is now, free to live healthy, breathe deeply and play with passion, your time is now (Willow, 2013).

Chapter 8

Acceptance and the Body

Taking responsibility for where you are in this moment

It is important to incorporate the body into the process of weight management and living a healthy lifestyle. You can soon see and feel that your body is not your enemy, it is your best friend. This chapter implements the **CARREZ** model (C – Commit, A – Accept, R – Respect, R – Reflect, E – Embrace, Z – Zone) which focuses on committing to action, accepting the present with respect, and then reflecting whilst embracing the new zone of thinking and doing. The **CARREZ** formula is explained in the 7 Life Steps.

The body plays an integral role because we need to accept and love the body, no matter what weight or size, so it can carry you through life the way that you want it to. When you take responsibility for where you are 'in this moment' you realise that you must take responsibility for what you may have inadvertently done at times to the body by overeating.

> My body is not my enemy, it is my best friend.

There is something really powerful about accepting where you are in the moment. All of us make choices in our lives. We choose who to spend time with, who to become friends with, what career or job to pursue and even what kind of life we want to live. We choose when to start and when to stop. Almost everything is a choice, except for our truly automatic bodily functions like our eyes blinking and our heart beating.

We also choose what we put into the body. Our choices make us unique, however our choices can also become problematic when we eat to satisfy an emotion or when we eat foods that do not support a healthy lifestyle. Often we search for motivational words, sentences and stories, or even people, to help us stay on track and keep the drive part of us stimulated. For this reason, Cas wanted to share a motivating poem that she wrote many years ago after she learnt so much about internal love and acceptance. Cas thought that the poem she wrote may be helpful and useful for those who at times have moments when they feel the need for extra support. You will notice as you read the poem that Cas focused on the growth and freedom she discovered as she grew up, including the inspirational aspects that flooded her with belief and determination to survive the world she was in, despite the lack of support and love. The poem is called 'Free to be me'.

Free to be me

As I was growing up, life seemed so huge and strange

As I saw the world, I knew that I would need to change

As I stumbled over my feet, my sister held my hand,

As I learnt about what I was supposed to do, I knew that I would need to be so true

As I was learning life's rules, I knew that I would need to be me

As I floated through the clouds of life, I struggled to be free

As I grew up, day by day, I learnt to trust

As I grew older, I learnt to distrust

Chapter 8
Acceptance and the Body

> As I learnt more about hurt and pain, I knew there was more to gain
>
> As I grew with such challenges, I knew I had the eyes to see
>
> As I grew older, I noticed things around me
>
> As I understood all that life presents, I knew that I had the sense
>
> As I grew more knowledgeable, I accepted what that would bring
>
> As I learnt to share my life, I knew that I could sing
>
> As I grew wiser, I learnt to share
>
> As I grew closer, I connected to people if I so dare
>
> As I stopped to hear, I listened to all that I could detect
>
> As I stopped to breathe, I noticed a voice deep down inside of me
>
> As I looked in the mirror, I saw all that was 'there'
>
> As I embrace the 'there' in me, I knew that it's okay to be so rare
>
> For I had forgotten that me was here, I soon realised I had nothing to fear
>
> Life is here and I am life, I knew then that I had chosen me to be free
>
> This is my life's choice and I am free to be me.

Loving yourself means to love all of the self, the mind, the body and spirit. The body is your sacred temple and you need to treat it with the utmost respect. It is so much easier emotionally to love yourself rather than abhor yourself. It does not really matter what size or shape you are, as long as you are on the road to better health.

Remember our saying?

> The object of this book is to help you live a healthy lifestyle permanently and to streamline the pathway of being healthy, living healthy, eating healthy, feeling healthy and thinking healthy.

You are THE most important person in your life. We know and understand that you may wish to be a good mother or father, husband, wife or partner, son or daughter, brother or sister. However, in order to be the best for others, you must first be the best person you can be for you, a form of selfishness if you like so you can be that best person for others. This process will take a mind shift and if you have reached this chapter, then you are ready.

An excellent way to demonstrate this theory is to imagine yourself out at sea on a boat, with small children. Now imagine the boat breaks down and you do not know how to fix it. You knew you were going out to sea with the children, who always seem to be hungry, so we now ask you, 'What will you do with the food that you have brought along?'

What is your answer?

Many people will instantly reply 'I would give it to the kids'. We then say, 'Now you are drifting, it is three or four days later. You have not taken any food and you are becoming weak, maybe even delirious. Who will look after the children if you are not strong enough?'

This brief exercise really brings home the importance of looking after yourself first, because in order to be the best possible person for others, you first need to be the best possible person you can be for yourself. The poem written by Virginia Satir, 'I Am Me' (1975), takes you on a journey of self-discovery, finding the true person within. The 'I Am Me' poem has been our pathway to help believe that internally we are what matters and what takes us to the next level of acceptance.

Chapter 8
Acceptance and the Body

> ## My Declaration of Self-Esteem
> ## I AM ME
>
> I am me. In all the world, there is no one else exactly like me. Everything that comes out of me is authentically mine because I alone choose it. I own everything about me: my body, my feelings, my mouth, my voice, all my actions, whether they be to others or to myself. I own my fantasies, my dreams, my hopes, my fears. I own all my triumphs and successes, all my failures and mistakes. Because I own all of me, I can become intimately acquainted with me. By so doing I can love me and be friendly with me in all my parts. I know there are aspects about myself that puzzle me, and other aspects that I do not know. But as long as I am friendly and loving to myself, I can courageously and hopefully look for solutions to the puzzles and for ways to find out more about me. However I look and sound, whatever I say and do, and whatever I think and feel at a given moment in time is authentically me. If later some parts of how I looked, sounded, thought and felt turned out to be unfitting, I can discard that which is unfitting, keep the rest, and invent something new for that which I discarded. I can see, hear, feel, think, say, and do.
> I have the tools to survive, to be close to others, to be productive, and to make sense and order out of the world of people and things outside of me.
> I own me, and therefore I can engineer me – I am me and I AM OKAY.
>
> by Virginia Satir
>
> (Satir, 1975)
>
> Used with permission of the Virginia Satir Global Network www.satirglobal.org. All rights reserved.

It is very important to love and respect the body because the body is your lifetime friend and companion, it is your vehicle to carry you and your soul and what you represent, including your thoughts and feelings, through this life. One of the keys to achieving a healthy weight is self-acceptance. We must learn to not compare ourselves to anyone else because each of us is different and unique. The most important body that matters to you is your own body. When we talk about loving the body, we do it in a different way because we may never really love all of us, we can love parts of us. Every little bit counts, as accepting the parts of us can only move you forward to accept what the body does for us each day. Instead 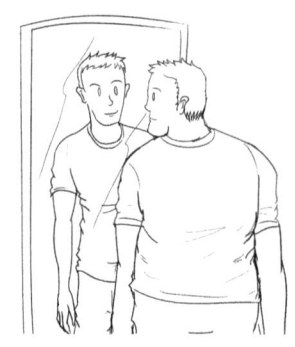 of looking in the mirror and criticising yourself for those little things you do not like, you can look in the mirror and love and appreciate yourself for those things you do like. This is a shift in perspective and a shift in thinking. We all have those little things that we do not care for when it comes to the body, however we would like to propose that you change your thinking. Instead of focusing on why you do not like a certain body part, why not focus on what you LOVE about that certain body part. If you find loving the body a little too different, then we suggest that you move into the thanking the body activity which follows.

> We cannot stress enough that acceptance is so important in this process.

Activity 19: Thanking the Body

Let's use the idea of our remote control once again. Every time you say something hurtful to the body like 'I don't like my hips or my legs' imagine yourself pushing that STOP button immediately. It really is that simple. After you push the STOP button, take a moment to quickly shift your perspective so that you can praise

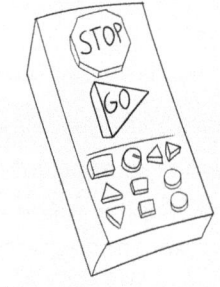

Chapter 8
Acceptance and the Body

> that body part. You can thank your legs for carrying you around and keeping you moving. You can imagine and thank the strong bones and muscles. You can thank the hips for supporting you, thank the nose for smelling, the eyes for seeing and appreciate what the body does do for you. Notice how the body works for us every day. When was the last time you thanked, praised and appreciated the body for the positives it is able to achieve for you every day? You can even praise the body if it does not work so well and, as a matter of fact, that is an even better reason to praise it. Encouragement is always beneficial. Then you can take the steps necessary to build upon the positives that you identify within yourself. Your body is doing whatever it needs to do the right thing by you. So being kind is a great start.

When you love the body internally and externally, you begin to appreciate the role that each part of the body plays in your life. Every part of the body is important, from the skin to all of the other organs and bones, right down to the tiniest blood vessel. This process is about respect for all parts of the body as well as respect for the mind. We cannot stress enough that acceptance is so important in this process. Remember that practise and even more practise can only increase the level of efficiency. The mind will make many mistakes along the way and it is important to recognise that it is okay and a natural part of being human. Just remember that when the mind makes a mistake, acknowledge it, and then move on to the next moment. We may not like some of the decisions we make, and it is just as important to ensure that you re-assess and make another decision to live the lifestyle you have chosen. All mistakes become part of the past – gather the learnings from them and move on.

Even if you find yourself criticising and judging your body, those other parts of you know that they are doing the best they can for you. Remember, validating how we feel about the body and how we see the body is the first step to appreciating the role of the body. Even if we do not love the body, we need to make the decision to respect the body and what the body does for us. This is a mind shift that can change your whole way of thinking about you.

The body is an incredible machine and vehicle serving us throughout our lives. It does so much for us, and we typically offer so little in return. You can choose to change that right now. You can start praising and appreciating the body for all the good intentions that float through each day.

You can and need to thank the body and the parts of the body every day for what they do for you, and doing so will help the transformative process. Remember, you made the decision to change, to do different. So doing different is here NOW.

We are all aware that to care for our bodies we need to eat healthy and exercise and be aware of what do we do for our minds. We continuously keep filling our minds with information and expect our minds to sort it out, without giving a thought to how we think and process the constant stream of information flowing into the mind.

Loving yourself NOW– no matter what shape or size

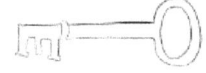

What would it feel like to love yourself NOW – no matter what shape or size you are currently? Loving yourself is a key. Making room or simply accepting yourself for who and what you are is also a key, alongside respecting and caring for self. It does not matter how much further you have to go; what does matter is how far you have come.

This process is a journey and you have already come a long way. By now, if you are following along and actually making the changes within yourself, you are gaining an awareness. You are changing how you look and feel from the inside out right now. You are transforming and shifting your perspective. The best thing you can do is to move into the acceptance of self, simply making room for self-views in this moment, and evaluate the progress you have already made.

Chapter 8
Acceptance and the Body

No matter what other people look like or what other people say, you are in the body you have right now and that body has come a long way on this journey. There may still be things you would like to change, just remember change is a process. For now, you are in this moment and you are what shape you are, so let's accept this and plan the future with goals and steps that you now live by, that will take you to the destination of your choice. Love and respect yourself for what you have and what you actually are right now.

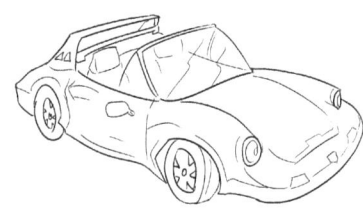

Remember, you are an amazing creation. You are incredible right now. You are uniquely YOU. It is time to be comfortable with who you are. You are not the body. The true essence of you comes from within, from the mind, the spirit and the soul. The body is your vehicle that carries the true and emotional you through your journey of life. Let's treat the vehicle with love and respect because you are worth it and deserve true balance in your life.

ACTIVITY 20: VALUES AND BELIEFS

Now take the time to fully understand your own values and beliefs. Ask yourself the questions: Are they true? Where did they come from? Are they useful? Are they helpful? Do I want them? Or will I change them? Be honest with your answers. We recommend you do this exercise alone. This is private. This is all about you and your innermost thoughts, feelings and beliefs, so it is important that they are not influenced by somebody else.

To assist you in discovering your own personal true values and beliefs and discovering what is really important to you, feel free to download our Core Values assessment sheet at www.CasWillow.com/Core_Values_Sheet.pdf.

Once you know what your true values and beliefs are you can set the goals to work towards ensuring that you are being congruent to your inner true self.

Appearance is a part of you, not all of you. It is an important part of the journey and discovering your appearance and your identity is vital for you to move forward. When you can appreciate and reflect on your positive qualities you begin to feel better. When you can put yourself in a healthier frame of mind by eating fresh, unprocessed healthy foods like fruits and vegetables, you just feel better about your choices. When you feel better you exercise and move the body more, which boosts your endorphins, the body's 'feel good' chemical.

When you love and respect yourself and think positive loving thoughts, you begin to embrace your own abilities. The body is only a small part of who you really are. When you stop comparing yourself and realise you have your own natural beauty and spirit, you realise that you can do and be ANYTHING that you want and choose.

Finding the motivation you need to move forward

We realise that at times it can still be challenging to stay motivated. In the end, motivation is really a choice, much like happiness. Just as you can make a choice to be happy, you can also make a choice to stay motivated. Feeding the body healthy foods supplies you with the energy to remain motivated; with more energy and motivation, positive results can be expected and obtained.

According to Harris (2010), motivation is part of a desired behaviour and is achieved when a person experiences positive feelings. The only down side to this is that when a person experiences negative feelings the motivational levels drop significantly, leaving a person not so motivated. Harris believes 'that if we equate motivation to a feeling, we will soon get stuck' (Harris R. , 2010, p. 229). Can you remember the last time you were so motivated that you felt on fire, focused and committed? Have a think about the drive to that motivation and see if you can recognise whether it was a feeling or a value. Then have a think about the last time you became quickly unmotivated, stopped what you were doing and just could not be bothered. You can soon identify what really drives you and what matters enough to stay motivated. Motivation works hand in hand with '**Choice Power**'. You make a choice based upon your true values to live the quality of life you have committed to thus far, and then apply the motivation pathway which will then become the drive power that you need to stay focused and committed. Often we can develop a lack of motivation when things become too hard or not purposeful. In order to keep growing and learning throughout life, work through the hardness and ensure that your focus is connected to a purpose. Motivation then comes to be a part of your desired behaviour that fits with your true values. You have the tools now to exert your **Choice Power** and be the person you choose to be.

Remember, all that you do now is your lifestyle change. You are making choices and changes that will stay with you for a lifetime. When you feel passionate and inspired there is no limit to what you can do. This often means making choices that are not always the easiest; however, it is about making choices of what is best. Often what is best may require a little more effort, just like climbing a hill to see the view takes more effort. The rewarding view simply cannot be admired if the effort to climb the hill is not undertaken. Everything has a process, so please acknowledge this and be patient with yourself and your personal progression, recognising that everyone is different and therefore processes will differ. Just focus on you and take the time to 'Note it' in your book or the NIB.

One of the best things you can do to stay focused and motivated is to start making small, consistent changes, one step at a time. Taking one step at a time brings you closer to your chosen destination. Make a commitment to move and exercise the body 3–5 times per week. We can sometimes lack motivation or enthusiasm and it simply may be because the body just needs to move and stretch. A brisk walk can and has the ability to release and relieve stress, so if you feel 'stuck' take a nice walk out in the fresh air. The brain releases powerful endorphins when you exercise and those endorphins, as you already know, are the body's own natural 'feel good' chemical so the body will search for many more.

Exercise and body movement do not have to be hard work; in fact, it can be easy, fun and enjoyable. The key factor is the intention of any body movement. It needs to be undertaken for the purpose of exercise. You do not have to go out and join a gym if gyms are not your thing or if you do not want to. You can simply turn on the music at home and dance around for 20–30 minutes per day. Some other simple ways to exercise are to walk up and down stairs, or using a chair stand up and sit down 20–30 times, holding in your core stomach muscles and not using the arms of the chair for leverage. Even after washing your hands having used the bathroom, place your hands on the vanity and do a few half stand up push-ups. Challenge yourself to be creative and think outside the box. Think about what you could do to move the body that is fun and acceptable to you. Just move the body to the rhythm of life. Moving your body to the everyday rhythm of life is a big step towards greater health. Do differently and think how you could be productive and creative with moving the body. Wiggle, shake, whatever you like; just move the body to the rhythm of life.

You can also meditate, do some deep calm breathing or join a cooking class to learn some new healthy, tasty recipes. Striving to learn new things can go a long way to motivating and stimulating yourself. If you commit to spending a few minutes in self-reflection mode every morning when you climb out of bed, you can hold in the mind the image of the new and healthy you. If all you have is five minutes, then that's okay because even five minutes is on the chosen pathway of self-awareness and self-reflection. Checking in with self is something we take for granted and often we need reminders to ensure that we are listening to the needs of our mind and body.

When we talk about change, we talk about doing different and doing different means moving out of what feels familiar to us into unknown territory. This whole moving out of familiar can cause some transitional issues. Being in the changing state can bring about awareness that you can become present within, without any interference from external sources. Change can be challenging because we are often comfortable where we are. This comfort can simply be because we are familiar and feel safe with the situation due to the fact that it is not the unknown. It is not always necessary to make huge changes, because that can be overwhelming and small steps to develop new lifetime habits are often the best approach. If you do not have time for an hour walk maybe consider going out for 10–15 minutes. You possibly spend at least that much time watching television or pottering with things that are not important, so instead why not spend it doing something healthy for the body.

It is important to remember that exercise does not have to be difficult. If you do not wish to join the gym or go out in the cold for a walk there are lots of simple and easy options, some of which you can do in the comfort of your own home:

1. You can put the music on and dance.
2. Using a chair, stand up and sit down without using the arms of the chair as leverage. Remember to hold in your core stomach muscles.
3. Do push-ups against the vanity basin after washing your hands.
4. Play on the WII Fit if you or the kids own one.
5. Play with your pets, they will love it.
6. Jump rope or jump on a mini trampoline.
7. Use a hula hoop.
8. Go swimming.
9. Play a team sport like basketball, soccer or volleyball.
10. Do some yoga or tai-chi.
11. Take a hike or nature walk.
12. Devise your own fun exercise circuit using objects within your home.

Body acceptance exercise

ACTIVITY 21: MOVING THE BODY

IMPORTANT! Stop right now and commit to yourself (not us) to move the body in some way, including in this commitment how long for and how often. Write this commitment in your NIB, diary, on a calendar, or even in your mobile phone with an alarm set to make sure you develop the habit. Motivate and focus on sticking to this commitment and resist making excuses for at least a period of twenty-one days. After the twenty-one day period you can be flexible and introduce new movement ideas, remember to continue to ensure you still have a commitment to yourself.

It may also be helpful to find some other like-minded people to help you stay motivated and focused, as there is often power in numbers. Congratulate yourself for how far you have come on this journey and give yourself a great big hug because you are more than worth it! Remember, living a healthy lifestyle is maintenance: maintenance needs to be carried out daily in order for the mind and the body to function effectively.

Let's do a little body acceptance exercise now.

ACTIVITY 22: BODY ACCEPTANCE

You may stop anywhere along the way to close your eyes, pause and reflect. You may choose to read each passage stopping to imagine the suggestions along the way, or you may read through the entire piece and then stop and reflect.

Begin by taking a deep and cleansing breath. Thank the breath for giving life and for nourishing you. Feel the breath moving through

Chapter 8
Acceptance and the Body

the body, cleansing and healing, to love and respect the body right here in this moment.

Thank the body right now and talk to the body with loving and respectful language and let the body know you appreciate it. Take stock of exactly where you are on this journey and praise yourself for all the work and the commitments you have made up to this point. By this stage, you have already made progress and the body is thankful. Notice the difference this makes, thanking the mind each step of the way.

Now rub the hands together to stimulate the energy. Notice how good it feels to use the hands in such a way. You may even notice a nice warm feeling starting to spread through the hands and arms. Take a moment to thank the arms for all that they do to help you care for the body. We hug people with our arms; they connect us to other people and to other things. The arms are strong and vital. They are constantly exposed to the sun and the air and yet they remain strong. Rub the hands up and down the arms and hug yourself, love and respect yourself.

Now stretch the arms above the body and notice how good it feels to release and ease any stress and tension. Feel the muscles and bones as you stretch. Thank the muscles and the bones for being so strong. Send love and respect to the body internally and send praise to all of the muscles, tendons, ligaments, the organs and even the blood. Without the movement of blood and fluid there would be no life. What an amazing body!

Now take the hands and rub them up and down the legs, noticing the strong muscles. The calves support us every day as we walk and move and they are incredibly strong. Thank the calves and the knees and the thighs for their hard work. Thank them and praise them and send them love and appreciation.

You might say something like: *'I respect you... I honour you... I love you. Thank you.'*

Feel the body responding to this love. The body does so much work for us every day.

Now take the hands and rub them on the face, feeling the skin and the lips. Notice how it feels to smile and be happy. There is no one else on earth exactly like you. You are incredible and you are unique. The face does so much for us, so take time to honour it and praise it. Thank the lips, the nose, the ears and the cheeks and thank the eyes for they are the windows to the soul. Our eyes are an integral part of our interpretation of all that we see.

Now imagine the back muscles and the stomach for a moment. The back helps the spine to support the body and carries us around every moment of every day and the stomach is constantly digesting and processing food. Thank the back and the stomach and the abdomen and all of the internal organs for all that they do for you.

You may want to just keep repeating: *'I praise you... I honour you... I love you. Thank you.'*

Bless every part of the body because the body gives you life. Honour and love the body every day for the contribution the body makes to you and your life.

Thank the brain for keeping you mentally sharp. Imagine how much it processes on a daily basis. We are nothing without the brain, so thank the brain for its service right now. Thank it for your intelligence, your humour and your personality.

Last, and certainly not least, thank the feet for carrying the body around. The feet are so important because they are the connection to the ground. Feel the feet on the ground and feel the earth

Chapter 8
Acceptance and the Body

beneath them. How wonderful are the feet to carry all of the body when they walk, run or dance, even for just simply being there, being part of the body.

Now let's thank any other part of the body you would like to thank if you are a woman, thank the womb because the womb makes you beautiful and lovely and supports life. If you are a male, thank the hormones and the testosterone, because they make you virile and strong.

Now just repeat in the mind until you feel that you have fully honoured the body for today: *'I respect you... I honour you... I love you. Thank you.'*

The body appreciates kindness. So tell the body you appreciate its fine work and its service. Tell the body you will always support it and love it. Apologise to the body for anything you may have done in the past that caused it harm.

Now hug the body and feel the power of self-love. You are incredible. You can do this. Every day in every way you are becoming better and better.

You may stay in this mode of appreciation and love for as long as you like and for as long as you need. You may do this simple meditation often or you may choose something similar on a regular basis to show yourself you appreciate yourself and that you are worthy.

If you wish, you may even choose to record this meditation of appreciation and play it back to yourself once, twice or several times per day.

Chapter 9

Setting Goals and Envisioning the NEW YOU

> Your goals come with plans or maps that guide you towards your chosen destiny, and destiny comes from your own creation and shaping according to your beliefs and values.

Setting the goals

Goal setting is an important part of any process and it is especially important in the weight management journey. You may know of, or have used, the **SMART** goals process, however if you do not know of it we have included a brief overview below that will assist you when utilising our program. A goal gives you direction and something to set your sights on, so it is essential for you to think through what kinds of goals are important for you as part of this process. Setting goals can be the major difference between the ideas and achieving the accomplishments because if there is no destination in mind, it may be difficult to begin the journey, stay focused and keep on the right track. Goals coupled with awareness give you focus and direction. They provide you with a plan for change as you make your way to a healthier lifestyle.

According to Stevens (2013), effective goals need to be specific and focused towards the desired result. Setting a **SMART** goal by utilising the following guidelines is the best way to stay on track and keep in check with your goal pathway (Stevens, 2013).

> A SMART goal is a goal that is specific, measurable, attainable, relevant and time bound (Stevens, 2013, p. 22).

'S' stands for Specific. When you strive to set a specific goal the end result is clearly distinct. You need to be able to state your goal in one or two simple sentences in terms of what you are looking to accomplish. This goal needs to reflect the state of mind or state of health you are looking to achieve. It is also helpful to state the goal in the present tense, as if you had already achieved that goal. An example of a specific goal would be '*I am a healthy and vibrant size*'. There is no need to always have to think in terms of weight, because sometimes stating your goal in terms of a size or being more healthier has more meaning.

'M' stands for Measurable. A measurable goal is one that has a specific target in mind. As part of this process, you ALWAYS want to focus on the state of health you are working towards, not the one you are moving away from. For example, it is helpful to state your goal in terms of the weight or size you are striving for as opposed to stating it in terms of the weight you are looking to 'lose' as we don't use this language anymore. Stating a measurable goal helps you focus in on the end result.

'A' stands for Attainable. In order for a goal to be effective, it needs to be challenging enough. Goals need to be challenging enough to make them a stretch and possible to achieve. It is important to ask yourself if your goal is realistic and achievable. Remember your focus is to stretch and grow and challenge yourself at least in some capacity.

'R' stands for Relevant. A relevant goal has meaning and purpose for YOU. You need to live by your own standards, as this is all about your life.

Chapter 9
Setting Goals and Envisioning the NEW YOU

Everyone has different goals because everyone is unique. It is important that your goal is fine-tuned to your specific needs.

'T' stands for Time Bound. For goals to be effective they need to have a timetable, otherwise they may not have relevance. Putting a timetable on your goal in terms of a specific date by which you are striving to achieve can go a long way to motivating you. Be generous with your time allocation to give yourself enough time to realistically achieve your goal and be aware of what you are looking to achieve.

Setting goals helps keep you accountable for your progress along the way and goals are a wonderful tool for motivation. Goals help you move from point A to point B and they are an important part of this process.

Achieving success requires you to have a certain vision of what that success looks like. When you break your goal down to very specific, measurable steps, you may find your goal much easier to achieve.

You can set goals for many things, including goals for physical fitness or for eating the right kinds of foods. For example, you might create a goal to commit to a brisk walk 4–5 times a week, starting out with a kilometre and working your way up to 4 or 5 kilometres. You could also create a goal to eat 3–4 fruits and vegetables each day. These types of goals are very specific, however, still reasonable enough that you can easily achieve them with a little effort.

> Goals are stepping stones to a result.

You can think of goals as stepping stones to a result. You are creating habits that support a healthy lifestyle and habits that you can adopt for life. You can create short-term goals and long-term goals because goals help you stay motivated and inspired. Your short-term goals are essentially the stepping stones towards your longer-term goals.

You can review and adjust the steps as you go along and as you make progress. Along the way, you may experience setbacks or obstacles because they are a normal part of any process. Everyone experiences impediments in life at one time or another and the key is to use them as learning opportunities.

Having thriving thought out goals can help you keep the mind focused because the mind always focuses on that which you continually hold in your thoughts.

> When you provide the body with a clearly defined roadmap, success is much more attainable and certainly more enjoyable, the body and mind need to know where you are going (Stevens, 2013).

The key to remember is that this process is all about healthy living and making those lifestyle changes that can set you up for life. When you provide the body with a clearly defined roadmap, results are measureable and therefore more likely attainable and certainly more enjoyable.

Goals are utilised in every aspect of life, including weight management, so learning to set **SMART** goals can help you in every area of life. Well-planned goals can help you turn thoughts into actions. While it is good to expand your thinking, you want to ensure that you are still maintaining good healthy habits because, as we have mentioned, this process is not about deprivation or starvation. It is about developing a healthy lifestyle, a lifestyle in which the mind and the body are united in what is right and healthy for you.

If you would like, take a moment now to create your **SMART** goal and record it for future usage.

Chapter 9
Setting Goals and Envisioning the NEW YOU

ACTIVITY 23: SMART GOAL

My smart goal for weight management and living a healthy lifestyle is:

_____

_____

_____

Sign and date here to hold yourself accountable:

_____

SMART GOAL: *A goal that is specific, measurable, attainable, relevant and time bound. Sounds easy because it is easy. Just be sure to utilise your* **Choice Power** *so you can be true to you.*

- What exactly do you want to accomplish?
- How will you know you have reached your goal?
- Does this goal require effort and commitment?
- Do you have the resources to achieve this goal? If yes, what are they? If you are unsure, what resources do you need?
- Is this goal one that is relevant for your life?
- When will this goal be achieved?

Now that you have set your **SMART** goal, the time is here to action it. Look back, reflect and make sure you have a clear and concise plan that can allow you to achieve this goal. We would like to suggest that you write this goal on a piece of coloured card using coloured markers and decorate it if you wish, making it appealing and motivating to you. Put this card in your wallet, purse or a significant place that matters to you. You see, these may be written words, however they are your written words, based on your human needs and your **Choice Power**, which you are now committing to action in your life.

Changing your self-image through future pacing

This process is much more than merely creating affirmations, learning about nutrition and setting **SMART** goals. It is also really important to change the way you look at yourself and change the way you feel about yourself. Visualisation is integral to this process because when you can see yourself achieving dreams and goals in the mind, you can easily change them from dreams to reality.

Taking the time to really focus on what you will look like, feel like and act like is the first step to making changes that last, because everything begins in the mind. Athletes use visualisation all of the time when they picture themselves making that perfect shot or winning the race.

We spoke about NLP earlier in Chapter 5 which went through an exercise to help with self-control. There is an NLP technique called 'future pacing' that is akin to mental imagery. It is designed to help you anchor in and connect the changes you are making to a future point in time. This kind of simple technique uses the idea of association and disassociation by helping you literally, or shall we say virtually, experience a new state of mind or a new healthy body.

What will you look like?

'Future pacing' allows you to experience a new body for size. The fact is that you can retrain the brain fairly easily by simply using your imagination. According to Cise (1994), self-reflective guided imagery amongst middle-aged obese women in a support group setting helped

Chapter 9
Setting Goals and Envisioning the NEW YOU

encourage the women to become more aware of the body and the mind in response to the environment. As the women became more aware of themselves, they began to fully understand how food and the past and present relationship to food created an impact on their current situation.

The women underwent a process that aided them to become in touch with their feelings and memories so that they could begin to process those feelings and memories. Cise (1994) stated, 'Obesity becomes the outward manifestation of the strategies used to manage troublesome emotions' (Cise, 1994, p. 177). In other words, Cise refers to obesity as being a symptom, not the actual problem, as many people unknowingly choose food to squash down emotions that they may have trouble dealing with or simply emotions that they feel the need to celebrate with. People who swallow emotions, as we refer to it, may find that their emotions come back with a vengeance. Cise also inferred that 'the body cannot tell the difference between an event that is actually occurring and one that is created in the imagination' (Cise, 1994, p. 180). What this means is that when you imagine yourself walking and talking in your new healthy, vibrant body, the body and the mind do not differentiate between reality and imagination. This is an incredible concept that can really change your life permanently. Once you learn to create all that you desire, you can then make it happen.

Another study undertaken by Kirsch (1996) found that the use of hypnotherapy could more than double the effects of a cognitive-behavioural treatment therapy modality. Kirsch also found that 'The data also indicate[d] that the impact of hypnosis increases over time, suggesting that it is especially useful for long-term maintenance of weight loss' (Kirsch, 1996).

These studies infer that mental imagery, whether or not it is used as part of hypnotherapy or self-reflective guided imagery sessions, can go a long way to assisting you to achieve the weight goals that you so desire.

When you really begin to imagine what it feels like to be the new you, the parts, mind and body have a clear direction in which to head. The more you use mental imagery, the quicker and faster you will manifest that new healthy body. Imagine yourself at the exact size and shape you wish to be and imagine wearing new clothing and standing in front of a mirror. You can even imagine yourself walking along a beach wearing a nice pair of shorts, feeling healthy and confident. The more you can be there in the mind, the faster this process manifests because the mind will find a way to make it so. 'Whatever the mind creates, the mind can heal and change' (Anonymous).

Imagine – what will you feel like?

How does it feel to step into a new healthy and vibrant body? Can you envision it? This is really a fun exercise because it allows you to road test a new healthier body. Imagine how incredible it feels to wake up in this new healthy body. Can you picture it? Can you feel it? Are you there in that new body? If you experience some difficulty with this exercise of seeing this body as a healthier version of yourself, simply allow the mind to create a sense or a feeling what your body may look like at the shape and size that you desire.

> The more you can imagine yourself looking, feeling and sounding great, the more the mind will move you towards this new you.

Notice what it really feels like deep down in your soul to be in this new state of health. Imagine that this was the one thing you no longer had to worry or obsess about. What would it feel like to simply eat healthy and think nothing of it? What would it feel like to buy the size of clothing you long to wear easily and effortlessly? What would it feel like to walk in this new body every day, feeling energised and inspired?

The more you can imagine and picture yourself looking and feeling great, the more the mind can move you towards this new you and towards that new healthy body. The most important aspect to remember is to continue to love, nurture and respect the body that you have right now,

Chapter 9
Setting Goals and Envisioning the NEW YOU

as it is the vehicle that has the ability to take you on this journey to your new destination.

> When you nurture your mind, body, and spirit, you then embrace the dimensions around you to expand into a new world full of adventures and experiences beyond what you have ever dreamed of.

Future pacing exercise – imagining the NEW YOU

ACTIVITY 24: IMAGINING THE NEW YOU

This exercise is designed to help you reflect upon your life and your state of health, wherever you happen to be.

You may stop anywhere along the way to close your eyes, pause and reflect. There are also suggested areas where you can stop and reflect. You may choose to read each passage stopping to imagine and notice the suggestions along the way, or you may read through the entire piece, as you desire.

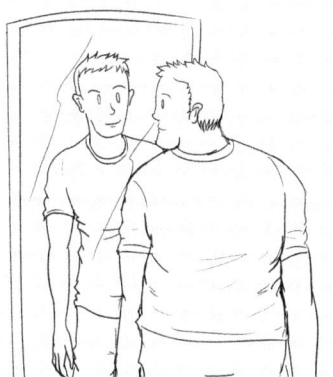

Future pacing exercise

Let's begin a little future pacing now. Begin by taking a few deep cleansing breaths. Just allow yourself to sink into relaxation and peace. Be one with the breath as it moves in and out of the body.

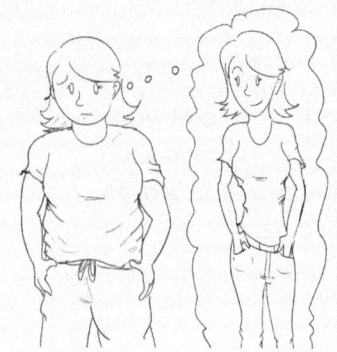

Continue breathing in and out, in and out until you feel a sense of peace and calmness spreading throughout the body. Continue to relax and breathe, and begin focusing on the type of healthy body you are striving towards throughout this process.

Ask yourself, in this very relaxed state of mind, to have a sense and a feeling of what a healthy body looks and feels like for YOU. This is about your ideal state of health so be clear to make sure this image is one you choose and feel a sense of satisfaction about.

Throughout this process you may either think of yourself in an improved state of health or think of someone you know that has the kind of healthy body you aspire to. This might be the body of a famous person, a body you used to have, or a healthier and leaner version of your own body.

Stop and Reflect...

Now begin by envisioning yourself standing in front of a three-way mirror. This mirror shows the body at its ideal state of health. You may either choose to stand in front of this mirror fully clothed or in something like a pair of shorts and a summer shirt, whatever you choose.

Think for a moment on that shape and size, your ideal weight. Now, in this very relaxed state of mind, your focus point is on the state of health you are working towards, not the state you are coming from. Focus on that ideal shape and size for you.

Stop and Reflect...

Chapter 9
Setting Goals and Envisioning the NEW YOU

You may take as long as you like to become comfortable with this process. Now allow yourself to see you transforming as you stand in front of this mirror. See the body shrinking and moulding into the shape and size that is right and healthy for you.

As you look into this mirror, see yourself becoming that which you aspire to, all that you have chosen to be. Continue to thank the mind and the body.

This is an effortless process because anything is possible with the power of the mind. Now repeat to yourself: '*I am now at my ideal shape and size, the size that is right and healthy for me.*'

As you look into this three-way mirror, notice how the body is changing, adjusting easily and smoothly.

Stop and Reflect...

Now take a spin in this three-way mirror. Notice how the muscles of the body are toned and tight. Notice how the stomach is flat and the thighs are slim. Notice how lean and powerful you look. You look and feel healthy and vibrant. Notice how much more energy you have.

You might even choose to run the hands up and down the body, feeling its powerful strength. Notice how firm everything feels. Take a deep breath in and notice how amazing you feel to be standing here in this vibrant state of health and wellness.

Stop and Reflect...

You know that everything you are or everything you can ever be is the result of those choices and decisions you make. If you want to change some aspect of your life, you simply need to make new choices and new decisions. It is also important to be committed on a conscious level and to follow through with those choices and decisions.

Now I want you to act as if you could literally step into this new body, this lean healthy vibrant body. Again, you can see this body as a healthier version of yourself or picture someone else's body.

Stop and Reflect...

Now stand up and actually see yourself stepping forward, into this new body. You could even unzip yourself from your old body and step into the new one just like you are trying on a wet suit. Now zip yourself into this new lean healthy body. Now notice how you feel being smaller and leaner. How does it feel to have already overcome this issue? Notice how you feel healthier. Notice how you feel more energetic and more vibrant. Notice if you feel excited.

Just keep envisioning yourself in this magic mirror at the ideal shape and size, moving around in this new healthy body. The more you focus on this, the more the mind can accept it as reality, slowly moving you towards this new reality, helping you make positive changes and healthier choices.

Stop and Reflect...

Now once you have become used to this new body style, see yourself moving out into the world with this new healthy shape and size going about your day. Notice how differently people treat you. Imagine yourself going through the motions of a typical day. What kind of food would you eat for lunch in this new healthy body? Notice how you make different choices? Feel how much you respect this new healthy body and feel the sense of pride.

Chapter 9
Setting Goals and Envisioning the NEW YOU

Feel what it really feels like... Deep down in your soul... **Notice how elated you feel and how amazing your life is, now that you have taken on this new body and this new way of thinking, moving and acting.**

Stop and Reflect...

As you contemplate this new way of being, you are moving into a new state of health, a new vibrant state.

You begin to really believe that you are capable of change, and it feels great.

Now imagine yourself in this new frame of mind, in this new healthy body just stepping into your new life, and feel the sense of freedom and elation. You might even choose to see yourself in a situation that you feel proud with this new healthy body.

See yourself walking along the beach or in a park wearing lightweight clothing. Feel yourself moving, running and jumping with ease. Notice how confident you feel. You feel so confident that you smile at passers-by, and they smile back. Everything feels easier, lighter and brighter in this new healthy lean body.

Stop and Reflect...

Ask yourself what kind of time frame you are working in now... Envision that a little time has gone by. You are living healthy, being healthy, eating healthy, feeling healthy and thinking healthy. Just keep practising how good it feels to be in this new vibrant state of health.

Take a moment now to allow the subconscious mind to imprint this new awareness as it transitions into a definite direction in your life's roadmap.

You may return to this place at any time to practise moving around in this new body, remembering to thank the body and thank the mind.

How did it feel to move around in this new healthy and lean body? The more you can imagine yourself looking and feeling great, the more the mind can move you towards this new goal.

Everything begins in the mind so it is important to see it, feel it, smell it, hear it and experience it with **ALL** of your senses. This new image of you is your role model and your goal. You might even cut out or print out pictures of people that have the type of healthy body you are striving towards.

Now visualise what you will really look like in this new healthy body. To assist you in this process, this is where we recommend you display that new item of clothing you purchased (or maybe even a whole outfit) with the store tags still intact. If you already have something in your wardrobe which has never been worn and still has the store tags attached, you may use this item. However, you must not have any memories associated with this item, as we have discussed previously. Remember to hang this item of clothing on the outside of your wardrobe and imagine yourself in it, every morning, every night and every time you happen to enter your room throughout your day. Make this as real as you possibly can.

Imagine you are at an event and imagine who else is attending. Be in the item of clothing and using all of your senses, see yourself, feel yourself, hear the comments others are making, notice and be in touch with yourself to really obtain a sense of how this new body functions in a healthy way.

Chapter 10

The Scanner

Learning to read the body's signals

In this chapter we will guide you through three different types of scanners:

- self awareness
- body senses
- the body scan

When you become more attuned to the body, you begin to understand and read the body's signals. The body knows when it is hungry and when it is satisfied, and it is the most reliable guide you have when it comes to food. We may tend to make a habit of piling our plates up with food without realising it or without asking the body what it really needs or even without 'checking in' with the stomach to see how much food it requires. We often allow ourselves to be influenced by what we think rather than listening to the signals and messages that we feel, of what our bodies actually need and not what our mind is telling us that our body needs.

Here is a little experiment for you. Close your eyes and imagine you are sitting down to a lovely meal. How do you know when you have had enough food? You cannot rely on the eyes to help you, so you must communicate with the body. You would have to ask the stomach when it has had enough. You would need to read the subtle signals the body gives you.

The mind and the body form a whole – you cannot have one without the other. There is power in just being aware, as the body communicates with you in many ways. It communicates with you through your appetite and food cravings, through your energy levels and even through your emotional and physical reactions and responses. We respond very quickly to the message and signal of pain. For example, if we have a sore foot we receive and respond very quickly to that signal to limp. This is due to the fact that our mind has a heightened awareness to pain and therefore responds very quickly. It is beneficial to our bodies and our health to adopt the same type of heightened awareness to all messages and signals the body relays to the mind.

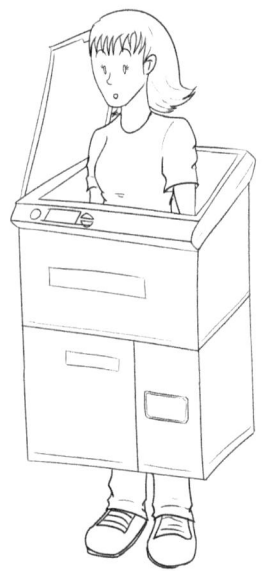

It is important to become more aware and comfortable with the signals that the body sends you and one way to assist this is to practise scanning the body. When you are feeling stressed or feeling hungry, you can actually undergo the body scanning process and learn to read the body's signals.

When you are feeling stressed, the body tends to respond. For example, the shoulders may tense up, the stomach may appear to be tied up in knots and the breathing may become shallow. You may also use a '**body scan**' to determine whether or not you are truly hungry or if there is another reason why you are reaching for food outside of a standard mealtime. When you are feeling hungry, where is it that you feel this hunger in the body? Are you hungry in the mind or is it the stomach? Does your body need fluids?

Appetites and food cravings are relatively easy to interpret. If you notice that you become hungry one or two hours after a meal, the body is telling you that your previous meal may not have been adequate. If your meal did not contain enough nutrients, or did not contain a healthy balance of nutrients, you may crave sweets, carbohydrates or other types of processed foods.

You can keep a journal of food and energy levels to check the body's energy levels and see if your energy differs as a result of the foods you have eaten. Ask yourself how your energy relates to your last meal. If you feel energetic and refreshed, then your meal was most likely a healthy and nutritious meal. If your energy feels drained and lethargic after your last meal, then the body may be telling you that the meal was not sufficient or it did not contain the proper balance of nutrients for you.

Checking in with your emotional well-being is also a great way to tell if the foods you are consuming affect you in a positive or negative manner. If you feel well-balanced, refuelled and restored after a meal then you have more than likely eaten correctly. Food needs to energise and uplift you, not drag you down, leaving you feeling heavy and lacking in energy. If you eat a meal and after that meal you feel sluggish, spacey or you are unable to hold your attention or focus, then the body is communicating once again, that it did not respond positively to your last meal.

ACTIVITY 25: TAPPING INTO SELF-AWARENESS

Stop for a moment and try this experiment. Close your eyes and start noticing how the body feels. You may choose to take a couple of deep breaths to clear the energy. Now ask yourself how you feel. Are you feeling satisfied? Are you feeling restless? Are you warm or cold? How do the hands feel? You can often tune in to stress and other ailments by tuning in to the body. The body carries stress and tension in the joints and muscles. Move the head around, from side to side and then forwards and backwards, and notice how good it feels. Now raise and lower the shoulders and notice how that feels.

You can even scan the body mentally and tune in to the body. Begin at the head and work your way down to the feet. Notice if you feel any tension or if there is tightness anywhere. Notice how the air moves around the body; notice your energy, and notice any areas that hold pain, discomfort or stiffness. If you reach an area that feels uncomfortable, sit with your energy for a while until you feel it easing. Ask yourself how you are feeling at the moment. Are you feeling stressed or relaxed? Happy or sad? Notice how your emotions have a direct effect on the body. Ask the body what it needs from you in order to feel better or more at ease. If you stumble upon an area that feels tight or concentrated, you can breathe into the area and send it healing energy. You can even gently massage the area and notice any sensations.

The **body scan** is a wonderful tool you can use to help identify any areas that may need more attention and it can be used as a tool to help gauge hunger.

The next time you feel hungry and it is not time for a meal, use the **body scan method** and see if you can tell what else the body may need besides food. Ask yourself what it is that you are really hungry for. Is it food or maybe something else on an emotional level? Scan the stomach and the digestive track to see if there is anything needed. Hunger is a physical reaction so if the stomach is actually growling, then you may need to provide it with some healthy options such as fruit or nuts or a snack high in fibre.

If the stomach is not growling, then it may be something emotional you are looking to fill. You may be bored, anxious, stressed or merely influenced by advertisements or marketing, which often tap

> into your senses utilising hypnotic or as marketers call it, subliminal messages, using the power of suggestion. If you are not truly hungry, then filling the body up with food is not what you need and will not be fulfilling to you. This is where you need to decide to take control and do something different, for example, taking a walk and breathing in some fresh air. Be mindful and aware of your decisions. Call a friend for emotional support, read a book, watch a movie, or undertake any activity that you know is relaxing for you. It is important to realise and recognise that you cannot fill an empty heart via your stomach. In other words, take control of you.

Learning to read the body's signals can go a long way to helping you in 'being healthy, living healthy, eating healthy, feeling healthy and thinking healthy'.

Being appreciative of the body

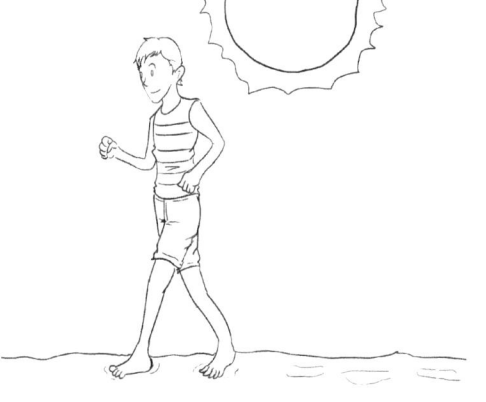

When you learn to tune in to the body, you can be more appreciative of the body. As we explored in Chapter 8, it is important to love and respect yourself in the here and now, for exactly who you are in this moment. When you provide the body what it needs for good health, you respect the body. Beginning to respect yourself starts the process of liking yourself, which helps with really understanding who you are and the differences you make in your life and others, which comes back to your values. Remember, we change our behaviours to suit our values and not just our feelings. When you take time to appreciate the body and thank the body for all that it does for you, the body repays you by giving you energy and vibrant health.

Gratitude can go a long way in helping you live a healthy life. When you take time to appreciate and respect the body, the body rewards you. The field of positive psychology tells us that an attitude of gratitude can help you to live the life you choose.

Research has shown that those who consistently practise feeling thankful and grateful actually have the advantage when it comes to good health (Krucik, 2013). Robert Emmons (2010), who is a psychology professor at the University of California in the United States of America, actually termed 'positive' psychology. His research found that people who adopt a gracious attitude as a permanent state of mind may, in fact, experience a multitude of health benefits (Emmons, 2010).

What this tells us as far as our work is concerned, is that there is a direct connection between how you feel and act and how the body responds. The research undertaken by Emmons and other fellow researchers suggests that grateful people:

- Take better care of the mind and body.
- Engage in more protective health behaviours.
- Tend to exercise more.
- Tend to have improved mental alertness.
- Are more likely to schedule regular health exams.
- Cope better with stress.
- Feel more optimistic.
- Have stronger immune systems (Emmons, 2010).

There are certainly many benefits from a simple practise like gratitude. Just imagine how the body can respond to a little love and gratitude if you take the time every day to express your appreciation!

Activating your other senses

When you close the eyes the other senses begin to take over. It has been theorised that blind people tend to have more acute hearing and other senses and it may just be the body's way of compensating. When you start to tune in to your other senses like sound, touch, taste and smell, you become more adept at using them. Here is another exercise utilising this practise.

ACTIVITY 26: TAPPING INTO THE SENSES

Close the eyes and begin imagining a bright yellow lemon. By closing the eyes you are instantly blocking out around 80% of the conscious mind. You are removing many of the distractions that clutter the conscious mind and using the power of the subconscious mind and the imagination, which can take you anywhere you want to go and you can be anything you want to be. Now obviously you cannot physically see the lemon, you may then imagine it. Now notice how bright the yellow is as you view this lemon. Now cut into the lemon and notice the juices flowing. Smell the lemon and how fresh it smells. Lemons have a very distinct scent. Touch the lemon and notice if the skin is rough or smooth. Now imagine tasting a small bite of the lemon and see how you feel. Move the tongue around inside the mouth, then notice and become aware of any sensations.

This is just one example of how the other senses become more acute when you begin to work with them. Notice the imagination and how it just worked with you and for you to imagine all of the senses engaging in that lemon story. If you really did follow those steps, it was real to you, was it not? The next time you sit down to a meal, take the time to really tune in to the body and the stomach and see what they need. If you are really hungry and it has been a while since your last meal, then the stomach will be communicating rather loudly that it is hungry and needs nutrition. If, on the other hand, you feel hungry and you recently consumed a meal, then you may need to stop and ask the body what else it may need instead.

The emotions are directly tied to the body and the body will always tell you what it wants and needs. (The time is now, to listen to those voices and messages which are numerous in the mind.)

The body scan exercise

Activity 27: The Body Scan

Once again you may stop anywhere along the way to close the eyes, pause and reflect. You may choose to read each passage stopping to imagine the suggestions along the way, or you may read through the entire piece and then stop and reflect.

Begin by taking a deep and cleansing breath. Thank the breath for giving you your life and for nourishing you. Feel the breath moving through the body, cleansing it and healing it. Begin to sense what the body needs or requires from you in this moment.

Thank the body right now and tell the body you love and appreciate it. Take stock of exactly where you are on this journey and praise yourself again for all the hard work and the commitments you have made to this point. Notice how the body responds to praise.

Begin breathing from the abdomen instead of the chest. Take long, slow, deep breaths and feel the body. Notice any sensations or feelings. Starting with the top of the head, and notice how the scalp feels. You may feel tingling or tightness or even a kind of energy flowing in from above. Now begin scanning the head. Do you feel tightness or do you feel a free flowing of energy? Notice any tension or any uncomfortable feelings. Sit for a moment and feel the energy swirling around the head. Now scan the face and the neck. How does the skin feel? Soft and supple or tight and drawn? If it feels tight or drawn tell the body you can take care of it by smoothing on lotion or face cream. You can even imagine doing this right now by imagining yourself in a healing pond or lake, splashing water on your face.

Now scan the shoulders and the upper back and the arms. How does the energy feel? Do you feel loose or tight? Breathe into any uncomfortable feelings and allow the breath to loosen up any tightness and as you slowly exhale, imagine releasing and exhaling those uncomfortable feelings, just let them gently leave with each breath that you exhale.

Focus on the feelings you feel as you scan through the body. Stay present in the moment and allow yourself some time in each area of the body, listening to the body and feeling the energy in and around the body.

Now move your awareness down to the lower back and hips. How does the energy feel here? As humans, we put a lot of stress on the lower back and hips so take a moment to thank the body, the back and the hips for the fine work they do. Scan the energy in this area and notice what you feel. Do you feel any areas that are uncomfortable? If so, sit with the area and breathe into the area and send the area love and gratitude.

Notice any feelings of tightness or pressure as you continue to work down through the body. Now scan the thighs and the legs. Do you feel any stiffness or tightness? When walking sometimes the muscles and tendons become noticeable. Again, breathe into any areas of concern or you may even massage these areas if you like. Or use the power of your imagination and imagine you are lying in your favourite place, and you are pampering yourself or being pampered just the way that is ideal for you. Allow your entire energy to just soften and lighten.

Next, scan the feet and the toes and see how they feel. Release any tension by wiggling the toes and moving the feet in a circle. Thank the body again for how it supports you every day. Send it love and appreciation.

Now make another full scan of the body seeing if the body feels different this time. Imagine you are sending a colour down through the body. This can be any colour. Begin at the top of the head with a bright and vibrant colour and notice how the colour changes as it moves down through the body.

Now send the colour out through the bottom of the feet and notice if it is still bright and vibrant or if it is dull or grey. Take this shower of light until you feel your energy clearing. Imagine you are out in the rainforest or your own favourite place somewhere in nature standing out in the sun and allow the shower of light to work through any areas of stress or strain.

Continue this practise until you feel better and more relaxed. Visualisation and imagination are very powerful tools and this exercise can work magic. The more you practise the body scan the more awareness you will have and the easier and more rewarding the exercise will be for you.

Chapter 11

The Remote Control

Dialling down your hunger

It would be fantastic if you could dial down your hunger using the power of the mind. Well, you can! The mind is a very powerful tool and you can use the mind to help control your hunger, and it is a very simple process.

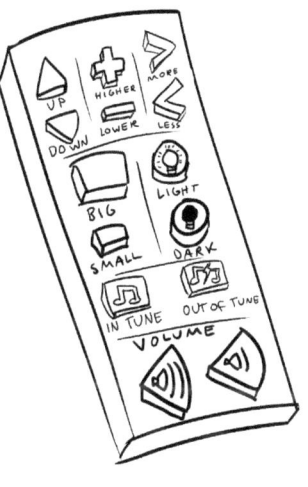

Just as you can use a remote control to change the channel on your television, you can also use it to control your appetite. Many times we mistake other things for hunger. The next time you feel hungry, stop and ask yourself if you are really truly hungry or if you are feeling something else. You may discover that you are thirsty, tired, depressed, anxious or even bored. Feelings can sometimes lead us to want to eat, however, food does nothing to help our emotions.

We like to use the analogy of a remote control to help with hunger. Everyone is familiar with a remote control, and it is something that is easy to imagine. Take a moment and imagine what your remote control would look like. This very special remote control has two buttons: a stop button and a go button. You are empowered to use this remote control whenever you like and whenever you need. You may picture any kind of colour you like for your remote control.

> You can use your remote control to adjust the screen and change the channel as you learn more about the stories that you might tell yourself as part of the hunger process.

This is a wonderful exercise to partake in when you feel hunger coming on and it is not time for a meal. We will delve further into the details of this in the remote control exercise, however, all that is required is that you can imagine yourself sitting in a comfortable lounge chair in front of the television. You can use your remote control to adjust the screen and change the channel as you learn more about the stories that you might tell yourself as part of the hunger process. Each channel takes you through your old stories within the mind, gathering your learnings to assist you in discovering how the mind and the body are connected.

The remote control assists you as you work through and analyse your old patterns and behaviours when it comes to food. When you come to a channel or an eating pattern or behaviour you would like to move away from, you can blur the channel, turn the volume down, scramble the channel, slow the motion down, or even adjust the picture from colour to black and white. This simple activity assists you as you work through the emotions and the feelings associated with food and behaviours that no longer work for you.

This is a very powerful activity that works effectively as demonstrated at the end of this chapter.

Chapter 11
The Remote Control

How do you know when you are really hungry?

So you might be asking yourself how you can truly know when and if you are really hungry. The stomach is approximately the size of a clenched fist, which is relatively small to what many people think it is. It does have the capacity to stretch, however 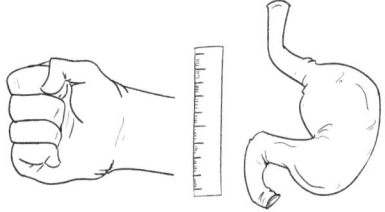 you certainly do not want to be stretching it every time you sit down to eat. It is really important to pay attention to portion sizes and to learn about the stomach and the body so you can learn how to read the body's signals. When you learn to listen to the signals and messages the stomach is giving you, it becomes much easier to manage your weight.

The next time you feel hungry and it is not a standard mealtime, ask yourself some simple questions:

1. 'When was the last time I ate?' If it was less than 2–3 hours ago, you may not really be that hungry.
2. 'Will a small nutritious meal or snack high in fibre suffice?' For example, you could choose to eat a piece of fruit and some nuts or seeds to satisfy your hunger.
3. 'Can I drink a glass of water and wait 20 minutes?' Sometimes you might find that you are really only thirsty.

If you are having trouble with hunger you might want to establish some regular times for meals and snacks, so that you are always prepared. Dividing larger meals into smaller more frequent meals is also a great way to keep your hunger at bay because you never quite arrive at the point that you are ravenously hungry. Also make a habit out of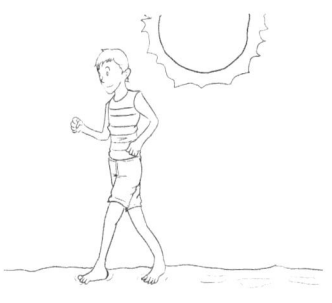

rating your hunger every time you sit down for a meal so you learn how the body works.

>  **ACTIVITY 28: WHERE ARE YOU NOW?**
> **Here is a scale you can use to gauge your hunger:**
>
> 0 – Salivating or ravenously hungry.
>
> 1 – Hungry with the stomach growling.
>
> 2 – Mildly hungry to the point that a light snack would most likely be sufficient. You could hold out a bit longer if you had to.
>
> 3 – You are satisfied and don't need to eat any more.
>
> 4 – You are more than satisfied and may have eaten too much.
>
> 5 – You feel like a Christmas turkey!

As we discussed in Chapter 2, ghrelin is a very powerful hunger hormone that stimulates short-term food intake and long-term body weight reduction. According to Zelman, ghrelin levels change profoundly in anorexia, in states of insulin resistance, in obesity and also, after bariatric surgery, suggesting that ghrelin is an important hormone when it comes to body weight regulation (Zelman, 2005).

Research also suggests that ghrelin levels are negatively correlated with the percentage of body fat and Body Mass Index (BMI), with findings indicating that ghrelin levels are actually lower in obese candidates that in those with normal body weight controls (Zelman, 2005).

So it seems from this that those who are obese might have a more difficult time when it comes to regulating hunger, however this does not mean that there is nothing that can be done about it, as the mind can accomplish anything it sets out to achieve. Whatever the mind creates, the mind can (if you choose to) heal and change. All of our patterns, habits and behaviours are learnt, so whatever is learnt can be changed if you are open to that change and ready, willing and able to make the adjustments that are required to make those changes in your life.

How do you know when you are satiated?

This is a great question as many of us struggle with this issue. In order to fully understand and recognise hunger signals, you have to stop and listen to the body so that you can understand when you are hungry and when you are full.

Hunger is actually a bodily sensation where the stomach growls and feels hungry, and it is controlled by many things, including a region of the brain called the hypothalamus, blood sugar levels, and even how empty the stomach and intestines currently stand (Health Care Registration, 2010).

Fullness is also referred to as 'satiety' which is a feeling of satisfaction. Certain nerves in the stomach send signals to the brain and tell it that the stomach is full. An increase in blood sugar, the activity of the hypothalamus and the presence of food in the intestines all contribute to this feeling of satiety (Higgins, Gueorguiev, & Korbonits, 2007). When was the last time you felt full or satisfied? What do you remember about those sensations? Do you really know when you have had enough? You will soon be able to know when you have had enough. This process will become easy and can be an everyday occurrence.

Appetite, on the other hand, has more to do with a desire or interest in food. The appetite can cause you to continue eating even after you feel full because appetite is linked with the sight, smell or thought of food and it can override both satiety and hunger (Higgins, Gueorguiev, & Korbonits, 2007). You are most likely familiar with the sensation of having no appetite even though you may seem hungry, which may happen during times of great stress or even illness. Appetite also, may cause you to eat even when you are not hungry, as in the case when you see an advertisement for a delicious food that you may be craving. We are often subjected to external factors that can contribute to our thoughts misleading the mind into thinking we are hungry and are in need to consume whatever it is we are seeing, in order to feel satisfied or fulfilled.

Dealing with hunger

When you take on the mindset of eating to refuel the body, you develop a much healthier approach. When you can separate eating from emotions and events, you will have a much easier time managing your weight, handling your hunger and living the healthy lifestyle that you have chosen.

> Eating slowly and mindfully, taking care to not eat in front of the television and eating at the table and really chewing your food will go a long way to helping you achieve your long-term goals.

When you really understand the true reason why you are eating and ask yourself if you are filling the stomach, the mouth or the mind, you will fully comprehend this process. Taking your time can help you enjoy your food more because you can enjoy the sensation of taste.

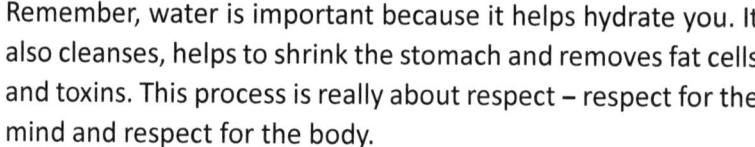

Remember, water is important because it helps hydrate you. It also cleanses, helps to shrink the stomach and removes fat cells and toxins. This process is really about respect – respect for the mind and respect for the body.

The remote control in action

Activity 28: Remote Control in Action

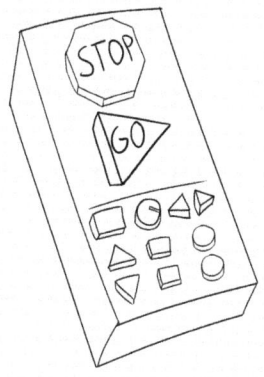

This exercise will help empower you whenever you are in a situation where the mind and the thoughts are leading you into doing things or engaging in behaviours that are not conducive to healthy weight management.

You may use this exercise anytime you need. The remote control allows you to look inside the mind so that you can see your stories. Many of us replay old stories in the mind when we find ourselves struggling with making healthy choices. We may think back to a time when we did not feel so great about ourselves and tell ourselves we are not good enough or deserving enough. If you or anybody else repeatedly tells you that you are fat, then that is the message that remains prominent. The great news is that you can change the message quite easily, all with the power of the mind and self-talk.

This exercise allows you to scroll through the channels of the mind so that you can analyse and discover the reasons why you might sabotage yourself. The **remote control** allows you to literally change the picture by either changing the colour, the sound, the volume or any other aspect of the picture you would like to change. You can either use a comfortable lounge chair in your own home or simply imagine one in the mind.

You may choose to read each passage stopping to visualise the suggestions along the way, or you may read through the entire piece, as you so desire.

The idea behind this exercise is that you can make good memories stronger and bad memories weaker. This is a really fun exercise to engage in as it allows you to use the power of the mind.

The thoughts and memories in the mind impact the way you feel. If you think about something depressing, you often feel depressed. If you think about something happy, you feel happy. In other words, you can make the happy memories even happier and you can downplay the sad or the painful memories. You can fade the old memories out, blur them or even turn them into black and white photos. You can make them larger or smaller, make them brighter or more colourful or even turn the picture into a static screen.

Most of us tend to think in one particular mode over another: visual or through sight, auditory or through sound, and Kinaesthetic or through touching or feeling. There are actually two additional modes which are not as common: olfactory or the sense of smell and gustatory or sense of taste.

Someone who processes information visually will see images in the mind when asked a question. If you process information in the auditory mode, you may hear certain sounds as opposed to seeing pictures. A kinaesthetic processor is more likely to feel emotions rather than hearing or seeing something. These three modalities could also be described as sight, sound and touch. Do not worry if this sounds difficult, because it is not. This will be a natural process once you begin the exercise and you will naturally gravitate towards one or the other.

For example, let us suppose that you have trouble with stress eating. You might think back to a time when you felt stressed and you turned to food for 'comfort'. By using the **remote control** exercise, you could change the picture and change the feelings. You could first imagine yourself engaging in the stress eating habit and then blur out the picture. You could also turn the colour picture into a black and white photo.

You can change how you react to stress in the picture and imagine yourself engaging in some other healthy behaviours as an outlet. You could picture yourself taking a brisk walk or drinking a cool, refreshing glass of water instead of eating unhealthy foods. You can also picture yourself eating a nice piece of fruit or even a bowl of popcorn as a healthy alternative. Now take this image of you eating healthy or an alternative behaviour as an outlet and brighten the colour and the sounds. Picture yourself feeling great about your choices and feeling pleased that you handled the situation in a more positive manner.

The remote control exercise

You may begin by taking a few deep and cleansing breaths. Just allow yourself to sink into relaxation and peace. Be one with the breath as it moves in and out of the body.

Continue breathing in and out, slowly and gently, until you feel a sense of peace and calm taking over.

Now you may imagine yourself sitting in a comfortable lounge chair. You can also imagine yourself in a room where you feel comfortable. This room has a large television in it, a very special television. Now imagine you are holding a large remote control in your hand. Your remote can be any colour you like. This remote has two buttons, a stop button and a go button.

Stop and Reflect...

Now as you sit in this room begin to review in the mind the thoughts you may be experiencing right now. Each channel on this television has a different picture. Think about all of the things you tell yourself pertaining to your weight management as you go through the channels. You might see channels that portray different images of you at different stages of your life. You may see yourself engaged in different stories or different scenes. You may use this exercise to browse through several different channels, stopping wherever you find the need. Simply use the remote control to stop and start at your own pace. As soon as you find a channel that you would like to analyse a little further, push the stop button and allow the picture to come into focus.

Now as you look at this picture, contemplate the possibilities as to why you might choose to overeat or make unhealthy choices, noticing what your mind is telling you about the picture.

Stop and Reflect...

What do you see on this channel? If it is something that is unhelpful or counterproductive, you can change the picture or change the scenery. You may also choose to do a number of different things including the following:

1. Change the colour to black and white.
2. Zoom in or out of the picture making it bigger or smaller.
3. Scramble or blur the picture so you can't see it.
4. Slow down the motion in the picture.
5. Quieten down the sound in the picture.
6. Change the picture in some way so that it portrays a more positive image.
7. Make the picture brighter or dimmer.

8. Sharpen the contrast.

9. Change the angle at which you view the picture.

10. Turn the picture into a movie and speed it up or slow it down.

11. Change the channel.

Experiment with this for a while until you become familiar with this process. The key to this exercise is to continue adjusting the picture until it looks exactly the way you intend it to look. Play with the sub-modalities like sight, sound and touch using the senses. You can have fun with this because the imagination is unlimited and you can create anything, any way you choose or desire it to be, utilising the power of the mind.

Stop and Reflect…

Now select another channel and play with this a little more. You can run through any scenario in the mind and work through any feelings you may be struggling with. The best part of this process is that you have the ultimate power to change the scene. Often you may have found you have given a word, thought or story more power than is necessary. It is important to realise you also possess the control to disempower the strength of that word, thought or story. This remote control exercise focuses on noticing that you have the power to change.

You can change the way you look at things and the way you feel about things. You can see yourself the way you want to be: 'Living healthy, being healthy, feeling healthy, eating healthy, and thinking healthy'. Continue changing the channel until you come to a channel that portrays you as you want to be. Feel free to use the imagination because there are no rules. You can reprogram the mind easily and effortlessly.

Know that whatever you want to create, you can create using the power of the mind. The more you practise this simple exercise, the easier it will be to adopt the changes you want and desire for yourself and your life.

Chapter 12

Self-Hypnosis Exercise

What is self-hypnosis versus hypnosis?

> Changing the way you think consciously and subconsciously can only bring about the change you want and you deserve to live the quality of life you choose.

Hypnosis is a common state of mind. We are hypnotised by marketing and advertising, by television, movies and even by the radio. Everything you have ever seen or done in your lifetime is absorbed into and recorded by the subconscious mind.

Self-hypnosis is really a very natural process and one you experience on a regular basis. It is that state of mind you experience right before falling asleep, that state of mind you experience when your mind drifts when you are bored, or when you are engrossed in a great movie.

The difference between self-hypnosis and hypnosis may surprise you. The truth is that all hypnosis is essentially self-hypnosis because each of us must allow ourselves to become hypnotised. One cannot be hypnotised against his or her will, no matter what you may have seen in the movies or on television.

It is a focused experience of attentional absorption that invites people to respond experientially on multiple levels to amplify and utilize their personal resources in a goal-directed fashion. Employed in the clinical contexts, hypnosis involves paying greater attention to the essential skills of using words and gestures in particular ways to achieve specific therapeutic outcomes, acknowledging and utilizing the many complex personal, interpersonal, and contextual factors that combine in varying degrees to influence client responsiveness (Yapko, 2012, p. 7).

Dr Michael D. Yapko is a clinical psychologist and a well-known author in the areas of psychotherapy, clinical applications and hypnosis. His professional life has been mostly focused on innovative treatments for depression. Yapko is also an international teacher who maintains an interest in the empowerment philosophy for clients to manage their own internal conflict and become their own master within.

Yapko (2012) says that self-hypnosis is something that everyone can do easily and smoothly and all you need to do is believe and allow the mind to do what it does naturally.

When you allow a practitioner to 'hypnotise' you, that is called hypnosis. When you develop the techniques and learn how to bring your own mind into that same state of focused relaxation, you are experiencing self-hypnosis. The advantage to seeing a professional counsellor, therapist or hypnotherapist is that you can dig a little deeper into the issue because the therapist can help gently guide the subconscious mind and challenge your current conscious belief systems.

A professional clinical hypnotherapist or ego state therapist has also trained in the techniques and has the skills to be able to assist you to drift into a deeper state of trance, however, with practise, it is possible to use self-hypnosis to make long-lasting changes. Self-hypnosis is a wonderful follow-up tool to use to keep the good work going and is often taught as a part of the session with the professional hypnotherapist to assist you with the utilisation of this skill in the future. Having said that, it

Chapter 12
Self-Hypnosis Exercise

is still possible to make changes initially yourself, simply by using self-hypnosis as a tool, assuming you take the practice seriously and remain committed.

When you undergo a process like hypnosis, you are using the subconscious mind to improve your life. The subconscious mind is where most of our information is stored and that information guides our lives. All of those little thoughts you think about and repeat day in and day out in the back of the mind rule your life.

Your thoughts become things so it pays to think positive. Many of us dwell on those things that aggravate or annoy us. If you continually tell yourself that you are unsuccessful, lazy or unmotivated to eat healthy, then that is what continues to manifest in your life.

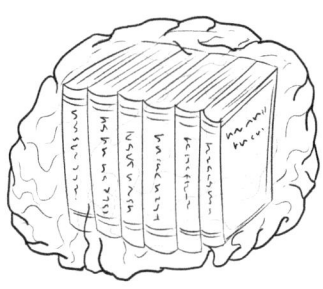

On the other hand, if you wake up every morning and tell yourself you are the picture of good health and you are living a healthy lifestyle, then that is what the mind brings into your reality.

Brief background of hypnosis

Hypnosis has been around for hundreds of years dating as far back as Ancient Egypt. The Egyptians used something called sleep temples to bring about a state of hypnotic trance and in many ways this was their form of a modern doctor. The Egyptians believed that the mind and body were linked and they used hypnosis, or rather an ancient form of it, to help bring about healing. The Greeks also used hypnosis in something called a healing shrine, which was based on the same principle as the sleep temples.

According to Yapko (2012), the history of hypnosis began long ago, even before we really knew that hypnosis existed. Hypnosis was utilised for the management of pain so that surgeries could be performed and patients did not have to suffer so much, as there was very little medically assisted pain control centuries ago.

> The medical use of hypnosis for managing pain has been well described for over 2 centuries. One particularly compelling narrative of the use of mesmerism is found in the work of James Esdaile (1805–1859), a Scottish surgeon serving in India in the mid-19th century before the introduction of chemical anaesthesia. Esdaile documented 345 major surgeries, including amputations, with hypnosis as the sole anaesthetic. These he described in his fascinating book *Mesmerism in India, and Its Practical Applications in Surgery and Medicine* (1846/2010; see also Kroger & Esdaile, 1957). Not only did Esdaile successfully perform surgeries that were extraordinary, such as the removal of 70-pound scrotal tumours with hypnosis alone, but also his patients had only a fraction of the complications (e.g., postsurgical infections, bleeding, mortality) that others performing similar surgeries had at that time (Yapko, 2012, p. 497).

Hypnotherapy has been used with dentistry as far back as the 19th century and the British Medical Association approved the use of hypnosis for anaesthesia for pain management in childbirth and surgery in 1955. Many people today tap into self-hypnosis when they attend appointments, such as visiting the dentist. Cas personally had suffered from a dentist phobia until she learnt and implemented the skills of self-hypnosis. She was able to allow her mind to drift into an Alpha state, often drifting into the Theta state whilst the dentist worked.

Milton Erickson, a 20th century therapist, completely changed the way hypnosis was seen and used by implementing persuasive language patterns as part of the hypnotic process. Erickson's usage of colourful metaphors and stories, as opposed to direct suggestion, led the way to further research into new and innovative techniques. Erickson believed that wherever you went with hypnosis within the mind, his voice would always follow to support and guide you through the process of healing (Erickson, 1982). Your own inner voice will take you there and guide you

Chapter 12
Self-Hypnosis Exercise

back to reality when you decide, within a set time period. All you need to do is let the mind do the work and allow approximately 10 or 20 minutes, then do the countdown sequence with peace and calmness. Do the self-hypnosis exercise in the coming pages and see how you go.

Whatever the history behind it, hypnosis is an amazing, incredible process. It has helped thousands of people overcome challenges and it can help you. With further clinical research it will gain even more credibility in the medical and scientific community going forward.

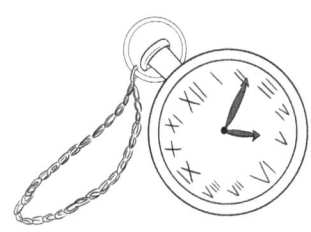

Brain wave frequencies – tapping into the Alpha state of mind

The mind travels in and out of different brainwave frequencies all of the time. The Alpha brainwave state is the state of mind often accessed during hypnotic trance. The Beta brainwave state, on the other hand, is the dominant state of mind most people are in during the course of the day. This is your conscious state of the mind which is filled with patterns, concentration, clarity, focus and being in the roused state. The Beta brainwave state corresponds to a frequency level of approximately 12 to 40 Hz. Harris (2002) refers to the Beta state as being the alert state which also sits in the '*flight* or *fight* response' mode (Harris B., 2002, p. 22).

The Alpha brainwave state corresponds to a frequency of about 8 to 12 Hz, which is a little slower than the Beta state. The Alpha brainwave state is often associated with a very peaceful state of mind, a state of mind very conducive to suggestion, which can continue to drift even deeper into the next state of the mind called the Theta state. Harris (2002) says the Alpha state has its very own way of moving into the relaxed and renewed state within the mind. The Alpha state continues to learn the pathway of finding peace and contentment.

The Theta brainwave state is much slower than both Alpha and Beta and it operates at around 4 to 8 Hz. Theta is a very deep state of relaxation or light sleep and Theta may also be accessed during meditation or deep levels of hypnosis. This state helps achieve changes deep within the mind due to its understanding level of creativity, memory and healing (Harris B. , 2002).

One of the slowest and deepest brainwave frequencies is Delta and it occurs around 0 to 4 Hz. Delta brainwave states usually occur in very deep sleep and this level of mind is not typically accessed during hypnosis. This is known to be the healing state which is vital for the body to heal, repair, flourish and refuel for the day ahead. Without the body and mind reaching this level regularly, the body and mind may start to produce complications with concentration, clarity, memory and may have difficulty managing day-to-day activities.

Accessing the Alpha brainwave state during hypnosis or self-hypnosis can assist you to make changes that can help you live your life in a more positive manner. This level is ample for you to achieve peace and the deep relaxation required to make the changes that you have committed into action through the creation of '**Choice Power**'.

The different brain waves are as follows:

Gamma Waves: Excited. Short-term intensity.

Beta Waves: Alert and working state. Concentration, arousal, alertness, cognition. Higher levels associated with anxiety, disease, and feelings of separation, fight or flight. Associated with worry, stress, paranoia, fear, moodiness and anger. Connected to weakened health and immune system. Fully awake and alert.

Alpha Waves: Relaxed and reflective state. Relaxation, super-learning, relaxed focus, light trance, increased serotonin production. Pre-sleep, pre-waking drowsiness, meditation, beginning of access to subconscious mind. Meditation and relaxation begins. Effortless creativity flows.

Chapter 12
Self-Hypnosis Exercise

Powerful state of memory and super-learning. A harmonious, peaceful state. Habits, fears and phobias begin to fade away; tranquillity and calm.

Theta Waves: Drowsy and meditative state. Asleep – dreaming sleep (REM Sleep). Increased production of catecholamines (vital for learning and memory), increased creativity. Integrative, emotional experiences, potential change in behaviour, increased retention of learnt material. Hypnagogic imagery, trance, deep meditative state, access to the subconscious mind. Insight, intuition, inspiration. Answers to important questions that are impacting upon your life can be found, great problem solving state. Feels like you are floating, feeling more connected.

Delta Waves: Deep Asleep – dreamless sleep. Human growth hormone released, often known as the healing state. Deep, trance-like, non-physical state, loss of body awareness. Access to subconscious mind. Healing and rejuvenation state, the best state for the immune system to function and restore health (Harris B. , 2002, pp. 21-23). Understanding the different states of consciousness and subconsciousness empowers those parts of the brain to act on what the body needs in order for the body to rest, heal and change. You have everything you need to enforce all that you desire both through conscious and subconscious brain connections to reach your chosen destiny. The following exercise takes you through the process of self-hypnosis so that you can regulate your own conscious and subconscious pathways within the brain. We have included self-hypnosis in this section as part of the linking process with the subconscious to bring about permanent change.

A simple self-hypnosis exercise

There are many ways in which to perform self-hypnosis. One of the easiest ways is to use what is called an eye-fixation induction method combined with a simple counting technique. The eye-fixation induction method helps focus the mind and it is very effective. Rolling the eyes upward and then closing the eyes sends a signal to the subconscious mind that it is time to go to sleep. This is a very simple technique that you can use as part of your self-hypnosis script.

Activity 30: Self Hypnosis
Let's start now!

Once again you may stop anywhere along the way to close the eyes and pause and reflect. You may choose to read each passage, stopping to imagine the suggestions along the way, or you may read through the entire piece and then stop and reflect.

Take a minute to relax and become comfortable. Find a quiet place to sit or lie down. This is your time to forget about anything that may be bothering you right now. Uncross the arms and legs.

Make sure you are warm and rest the hands loosely in the lap and take a long, slow deep breath, feeling the breath as it enters the body and becomes warm as it gently travels down into the lungs, holding the breath in for just a moment.

As you exhale, feel the body releasing toxins, stress and negativity. Now focus the eyes on something above the head, perhaps on a spot on the wall or the ceiling so the eyes are strained just a bit. Keep them that way, as long as you can, slowly counting backwards from 100. This kind of eyestrain, once you finally close the eyes, puts you into a nice light level of hypnosis. Do not worry if you become tired and do not want to finish counting backwards; that is the idea. Just allow the numbers to drift right on out of the mind.

You may also imagine you are writing each number up on a chalkboard then erasing and writing the next number. Slowly begin counting backwards until the mind drifts and the intention to continue counting fades. Notice as you count that the eyes will begin to feel strained and begin to water. Keep them open for as long as you can.

Chapter 12
Self-Hypnosis Exercise

100... 99... 98... 97... 96... 95... 94... 93... 92... 91... etc.

As you count backwards, continue breathing deeply... holding in the breath for just a moment, before slowly exhaling as you empty the lungs completely, releasing all remaining tension and stiffness. Take another deep breath, as you continue to count backwards, and gently exhale, allowing yourself to drift into a state of deep relaxation.

When you come to the point where you cannot keep the eyes open, close them gently as you let your attention drift.

You may either give yourself some positive suggestions or simply relax, drift and dream. If you do not have your suggestions memorised, simply open the eyes and read them, then close the eyes again, continuing to relax. We have included affirmations, as the mind requires the directional pathways and the belief that you are serious about what you are doing. Affirmations, utilised wisely, empower those parts of the brain to activate the learning process and bring about the required change.

You can utilise affirmations as mantras if you so choose. According to Chopra, a well-known author in the spiritual and meditative realm, the word:

> mantra has two parts: 'man,' which in Sanskrit means 'mind,' and 'tra,' which means 'instrument.' A mantra is therefore an instrument of the mind, a powerful sound or vibration that you can use to enter a deep state of meditation. Silently repeating a mantra as you meditate is a powerful way to enter the silence of the mind. As you repeat the mantra, it creates a mental vibration that allows the mind to experience deeper levels of awareness. The mantra then becomes increasingly abstract and indistinct, until you're finally led into the field of pure consciousness from which the vibration arose – your spirit (Chopra, 2013).

A mantra is something that you believe in and repeat over and over again, 20–30 times per day or even more. A mantra allows for the words to float through into a deeper level to bring about the desired effect. This is how it can work for you. You can choose one line of the affirmation and then repeat it over and over again to a hum or a tune that uplifts you.

Example: 'I'm free to be me, I'm free to be me, I'm free to be me, I'm free to be me.' Embrace the feeling that flows from the mantra and embrace the sensation of vibrations that may linger within the body. Mantras are a powerful tool to increase self-worth and self-awareness.

Activity 31: Weight Management Affirmations

Here are some simple weight management suggestions you can use. Repeat them aloud or tape them for you to hear them in your own voice.

1. I am living healthy, eating healthy, feeling healthy, being healthy and thinking healthy.
2. I love living a healthy lifestyle.
3. I choose to be free.
4. I have choices in my life.
5. I take responsibility for what I do and say.
6. I am me, all of me and I choose to _____
7. I enjoy finding new and creative ways to exercise and move the body.
8. I am healthier and leaner every day.
9. As I am healthier, my energy increases.

Chapter 12
Self-Hypnosis Exercise

10. I have a naturally high metabolism.
11. My fat drips away as I throw away extra weight.
12. I easily let go of anything and everything that does not support me.
13. I am proud and confident.
14. Food is fuel for the engine that is the body.
15. I eat healthy, nutritious foods in just the right amounts.
16. I eat my food slowly, chewing it thoroughly.
17. Healthy foods are delicious foods.
18. I enjoy eating real, clean, natural, nutritious or fresh unprocessed foods.
19. I am the picture of good health and it shows.
20. I live my life through new lenses.

Tell yourself that these suggestions are now firmly and deeply embedded within the subconscious mind where they will grow stronger and stronger each day.

Ask yourself what kind of time frame you are working in now... Envision that a little time has gone by. You have won the battle and overcome much. You are living, eating, being, feeling and thinking healthy. Just keep practising how good it feels to be in this new vibrant state of health.

Now imagine moving around in this leaner and healthier body. The more you can imagine yourself looking and feeling great, the more the mind will move you towards this new goal.

Everything begins in the mind, so it is important to see it, feel it and experience it with all of your senses. This new image of you is your role model and your goal.

> Imagine visualising what you really look like in this new healthy body. Imagine an image of yourself enjoying this new leaner body, shopping for smaller clothes, or eating lunch with friends, not having to be so self-conscious of what you eat and not feeling judged by what they must be thinking about you.
>
> Imagine feeling what it is like to have a new positive, helpful and confident attitude about the body. Now imagine yourself chatting with someone about how you reached this important goal. What are you saying about your success? Imagine how confident you feel showing yourself off. Notice how the people around you respond.
>
> Using your senses, really see what you see, feel what you feel and hear what you hear, as you become in touch with yourself to gain a sense of how this new body works.
>
> Now take a moment to envision yourself six months down the track. Notice how different you are in this new state of mind. Stay in this visualisation as long as you like and as long as you need.
>
> When you are finished, you can simply count yourself up from 1 to 5.

The following checklist is called **CRAN** (as described in step 7), the safeguard system: Check, Reflect, Adjust and Nurture. The **CRAN** is there as part of the maintenance program to ensure that you have everything you need for your body and mind to continue to run smoothly just like the car you have chosen, to carry you through life.

We start the process by checking where you are *AT* right now, what is happening for you? Are you where you want to be? Are you doing what you choose to do according to your values and beliefs? If you need to adjust anything, then add that to the box, and then nurture self to ensure you have accepted the adjustment. We suggest weekly to monthly **CRANs** at first and then, once you are living a healthy lifestyle, you can follow the **CRAN** according to your needs once you have the pattern in place.

Chapter 12
Self-Hypnosis Exercise

 **ACTIVITY 32: THE CRAN CHECKLIST: THE SAFEGUARD SYSTEM**

Apply Preservation Process

C = Check
- Q. _____
- Q. _____
- Q. _____
- Q. _____

R = Reflect
- Q. _____
- Q. _____
- Q. _____
- Q. _____

A = Adjust

[   ]

N = Nurture
_____
_____
_____

Conclusion

Congratulations!

You are now living healthy, eating healthy, feeling healthy, being healthy and thinking healthy.

You have come a long way on this journey and you have made a lot of progress. By now you know that 'diets' are not an effective long-term solution because they never actually address the core of the issues behind why the weight is there in the first place. As we mentioned in the beginning, the object of this book is to help streamline the pathway of being, living, eating, feeling and thinking healthy.

In order for the weight to drip away, there is a part of you, or perhaps many parts of you, that needed and wanted to change. You have worked on all of those parts of you and the whole you as you have made your way through this book and this process.

We recommend you go back through and repeat any of the exercises that you found most helpful and useful for you. When in doubt or if things are not flowing as you believe they ought to for you, simply go back and check the basics. Ask yourself, what is it that you are not putting into practise; it will be something simple that you are overlooking. This book is all about changing the way you think, look and feel by helping you learn about your relationship with food. Food is not the enemy and it is not necessary to starve yourself. As you have travelled on this journey with us, we trust you now have a greater appreciation and respect for the body and for the amazing creation and work of art that it is. 'You are your own masterpiece, your own creation, filled with unique qualities, extraordinary differences that create your self-power to be your own authority of the mind. Let no-one take that away from you' (Willow, 2011).

When you practise techniques like mindful eating, you are present in the moment and very aware of the decisions you make on a conscious level. When you eat foods that are healthy and nutritious you feel more energised. Think about that term 'healthy lifestyle' again. Do you view this term differently now that you have read this book? You most likely see yourself in a new light. When you live a healthy lifestyle, you no longer have to continually fret and fuss over food. You can eat what you love in healthy portions when you choose foods that are healthy and nutritious.

Life is meant to be enjoyed not just endured. One of our goals that we wished for you was to provide you with all the tools that you needed to gain control over your life as it pertains to weight management. If you take away only one aspect from this, we trust that you have learnt that it is important to love and respect yourself, regardless of the situation. It is important for you not to compare yourself to anyone else, because each of us has our own unique qualities and beauty.

We have enjoyed writing and sharing our journey and this process with you. If you need any further assistance, please feel free to contact us or your local qualified counsellor or clinical hypnotherapist who specialises in the CaS Therapy Weight Management and Lifestyle techniques and who practise any of the techniques shared with you on this journey.

> Dance like nobody's watching;
> love like you've never been hurt.
> Sing like nobody's listening;
> live like it's heaven on earth.
> Mark Twain

We wish you every success as you travel on the road through the journey of life that lies ahead. You have the choice which vehicle you drive, and to some degree (naturally there are some things that are beyond your control) you have the choice as to the condition that vehicle is in when you arrive at that destination, so remember to tune in to that inner voice that speaks to you. 'Hey, Hey It's Me.' Remember, you are truly amazing.

Conclusion

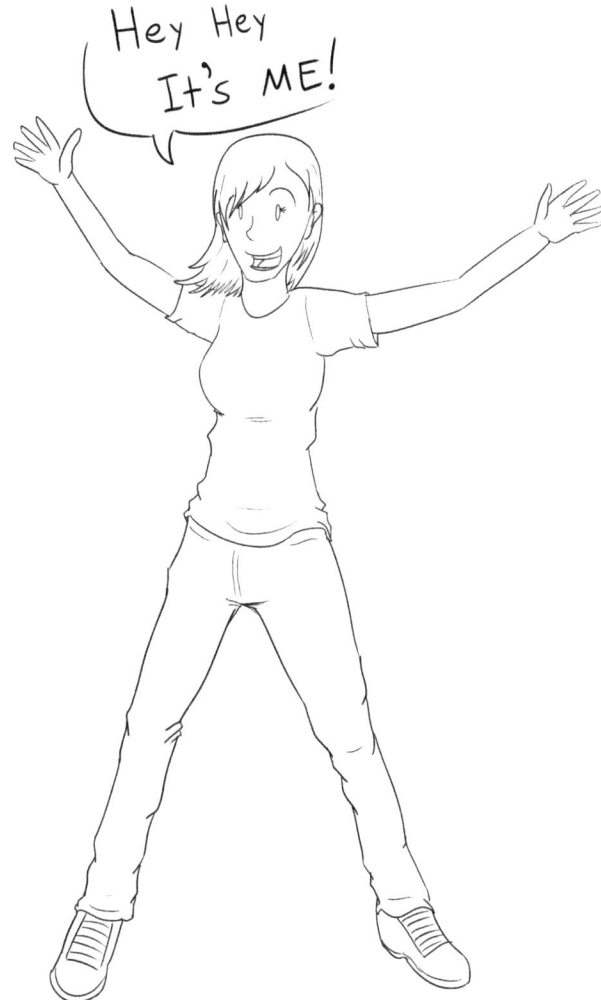

Congratulations, you have made it through to

'The End'

of the book, however it is the beginning of the new you if you choose it to be.

References

Albers, S. P. (2012). *Eating mindfully: How to end mindless eating and enjoy a balanced relationship with food.* Oakland, California: New Harbinger Publications, Inc.

Appleton, PhD, N., & Jacobs, G. N. (2009). *Suicide by sugar.* Garden City Park, New York, United States of America: Square One Publishers.

Baer, R. A. (2006). Mindfulness-based treatment approaches. (R. A. Baer, Ed.) Burlington, United States of America: Elsevier Acedemic Press. Retrieved January 13, 2014, from http://www.scribd.com/doc/69423170/Mindfulness-Based-Treatment-Approaches-Baer-2006

Bandler, R., & Grinder, J. (1975). *The structure of magic.* California, Palo Alto: Science and Behavior Books Inc.

Barnett, S. (2006). *Calm.* Kansas City, Missouri: Andrews McMeel.

CaSandH Pty. Ltd. (2010, February 13). *Hypnotherapy*. Retrieved November 9, 2013, from CaS Therapy: http://www.caswillow.com/services/a-bit-about-hypnotherapy/#sthash.HSpbuT3a.dpuf

CaSandh Pty. Ltd., & Richards, H. G. (2010, February 13). *Ego State Therapy*. Retrieved November 9, 2013, from Cas Therapy: http://www.caswillow.com/services/ego-state-therapy/#sthash.bWayOhhl.dpuf

Chopra. (2013). *What is a Mantra?* (Chopra Centre) Retrieved April 11, 2014, from Chopra Centre of Meditation: http://www.chopra.com/ccl-meditation/21dmc/mantra.html

Cise, J. C. (1994). Self-reflective guided imagery among middle-aged obese women in a support group setting. (Order No. 9519613, Indiana

Univeristy School of Nursing). Retrieved November 10, 2013, from http://search.proquest.com/docview/304166651?accountid=458. (prod.academic_MSTAR_304166651).

Edelman, S. (2006). *Change your thinking.* Sydney, New South Wales: ABC Books.

Emmerson, G. (2009). *Ego state therapy.* Bethel, United States of America: Crown House Publishing.

Emmons, R. (2010, November 16). *Why Gratitude is Good*. Retrieved November 10, 2013, from Greater Good: http://greatergood.berkeley.edu/article/item/why_gratitude_is_good

Erickson, M. H. (1982). *My voice will go with you:The teachings tales of Milton H. Erickson.* (S. Rosen, Ed.) New York, United States of America: Norton.

Fahey, T. D., Insel, P. M., & Roth, W. T. (2010). *Looking Ahead*. Retrieved January 25, 2014, from Nutrition Chapter 8: http://highered.mcgraw-hill.com/sites/dl/free/0078022584/947562/SampleChapter08.pdf

Fred, L. (2001, May 15). *Ivan Petrovich Pavlov (1849-1936)*. Retrieved November 10, 2013, from Nobel Proze.org: The offical website of the nobel proze: http://www.nobelprize.org/educational/medicine/pavlov/readmore.html

Furlonger, B. (2013). *Introduction to counselling across the lifespan.* Monash University: Faculty of Education.

Geldard, D., & Geldard, K. (2012). *Basic personal counselling* (7 ed.). New South Wales: Pearson Australia.

Glasser, W. M. (1998). *Choice theory.* New York, United States of America: HarperCollins Publishers.

Glasser, W. M. (2000). *Reality therapy in action.* New York, United States of America: Harpercollins Books.

Gray, J. (2003). *The mars & venus diet & excercise solution.* New York, United States of America: Martin's Press.

Harris, B. (2002). *Thresholds of the mind.* Oregan, United States of America: Centrepointe Press.

Harris, R. (2007). *The happiness trap.* New South Wales, Australia: Exislepublishing.

Harris, R. (2007). *The happiness trap.* Retrieved November 10, 2013, from http://www.thehappinesstrapcom/about.

Harris, R. (2009). *ACT made simple.* Oakland, United States of America: New Harbinger.

Harris, R. (2010). *The confidence gap, from fear to freedom.* London, England: Peguin Books Ltd.

Hayes, S. (2004). Acceptance and commitment therapy, relational frame theory, and the third wave of behavioral and cognitive therapies. *Behavior Therapy, 35*, 639-665. Retrieved November 9, 2013

Hayes, S. C., & Smith, S. (2005). *Get out of your mind and into your life.* Oakland, Unites States of America: New Harbinger.

Health Care Registration. (2010). *Effective GoalSetting, 19, 12.*

Higgins, S., Gueorguiev, M., & Korbonits, M. (2007). Ghrelin, the peripheral hynger hormone. *Annals Of Medicine*, 39(2), 116-126.

Kirsch, I. (1996). Hypnotic enhancement of cognitive-behavioral weight loss treatments:Another meta-reanalysis. *Journal of Consulting and Clinical Psychology*, 64(3), 517-519. doi:doi:http://dx.doi.org/10.1037/0022-006X.64.3. Page 519.

Krucik, G. M. (2013). *A Dose of Gratitude: How Being Thankful Can Keep You Healthy*. (R. Madell, Editor) Retrieved November 9, 2013, from Healthline.

Lao-tzu. (2013). *Quotations by Author*. Retrieved November 8, 2013, from The Quotation Page: http://www.quotationspage.com/quotes/Lao-tzu/

Medicine, J. H. (2007). *The Dangers of too much body fat*. Retrieved November 10, 2013, from Johns Hopkins Health Alert: http://www.johnshopkinshealthalerts.com/alerts/nutrition_weight_control/JohnsHopkinsHealthAlertsNutritionWeightControl_813-1.html

Mindful eating. (2011). *Harvard Health Letter,* (3), 36.

NaturalNews. (2012, August 08). *Interview with Don Tolman. the Whole Food Medicine Cowboy*. Retrieved November 9, 2013, from Natural Health News & Scientific Discoveries: http://www.naturalnews.com/036728_Don_Tolman_Whole_Food_Medicine_Cowboy_interview.html#ixzz2bre0sjfo.

Ostrow, R. (2007). *Life magic*. Australia, Victoria: Hardie Grant Books.

Park, G. (2009). *7 secrets the weight loss industry will never tell you*. Queensland, Austalia: AWL PTY Limited.

Satir, V. (1975). *Self-Esteem*. Retrieved January 26, 2014, from http://members.shaw.ca/strive4balance/satir.html

Shurkin, J. N. (2004). Eating to live longer. *Time Inc. Health*, 132-136.

Sifferlin, A. (2013, June 28). *What makes shakes teach us about food addiction*. Retrieved November 9, 2013, from CNN Time: http://www.cnn.com/2013/06/28/health/time-food-addiction

Stevens, A. (2013). *Turn your dreams and wants into achievable smart goals.* Anna Stevens, EQ for Success LLC.

Wansink, B. (2010). *Mindless eating.* New York, United States of America: Bantam Books.

Wayant, P. (2005). *Think positive thoughts everyday.* United States of America: Blue Mountain Press.

Weil, A. (2007, August 27). Mindful eating key to healthy eating. *Edmonton*. Retrieved December 3, 2013, from http://search.proquest.com/docview/253466059?accountid=458

Williamson, M. (n.d.). *A Year of Miracles*. Retrieved December 3, 2013, from Marianne Williamson: http://www.marianne.com/

Yapko, M. M. (2012). *Trancework* (4 ed.). New York, United States of America: Routledge.

Zelman, K. M. (2005). *Weight Loss and Diet Plans*. Retrieved January 27, 2014, from WebMD: http://www.webmd.com/diet/features/really-hungry

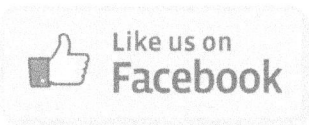

If you are enjoying your journey through the book and would like to get to know us and join the "Hey Hey It's Me!" online social media community, then please do "Like us" and share your experience with others and with your friends.

Getting to Know Us on Facebook

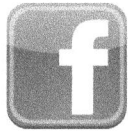

www.Facebook.com/HeyHeyItsMeWeightManagement

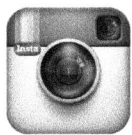

we are on Instagram as CaS Therapy:

http://instagram.com/castherapy/

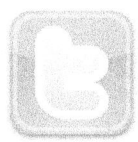

on Twitter follow Heather: https://twitter.com/HeatherRichards

or simple visit our blog

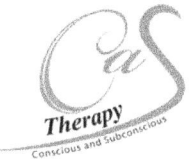

http://www.CasWillow.com/Whats-News/

FEEL FREE to email your questions to

CasandHeather@HeyHeyItsMe.com or
if you wish to share publicly, then join our online community.

QR-CODES

www.CasWillow.com/whats-news

www.HeyHeyItsMe.com

www.CasWillow.com

www.HypnoticGastricBanding.com

www.ingramcontent.com/pod-product-compliance
Ingram Content Group UK Ltd.
Pitfield, Milton Keynes, MK11 3LW, UK
UKHW021313180426
11947UKWH00015B/1207